HEALTH & WEIGHT-LOSS
BREAKTHROUGHS
2009

NEWS YOU
CAN USE NOW!

FROM THE EDITORS OF **Prevention.**

RODALE

© 2009 by Rodale Inc.

All rights reserved. No part of this publication may be reproduced or transmitted in any form or by any means, electronic or mechanical, including photocopying, recording, or any other information storage and retrieval system, without the written permission of the publisher.

Prevention is a registered trademark of Rodale Inc.

Printed in the United States of America
Rodale Inc. makes every effort to use acid-free ♾, recycled paper ♻.

Book design by Carol Angstadt
Photograph Credits can be found on page 334.

ISBN-13 978–1–60529–975–4
ISBN-10 1–60529–975–8

2   4   6   8   10   9   7   5   3   1   hardcover

We inspire and enable people to improve their lives and the world around them
For more of our products visit **rodalestore.com** or call 800-848-4735

CONTENTS

PART I:
HEALTH BREAKTHROUGHS

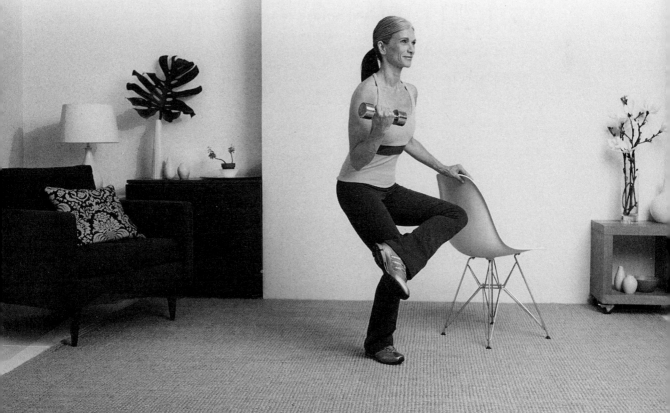

PART II:
NUTRITION NEWS

PART III:
WEIGHT-LOSS WISDOM

PART IV:
FITNESS TRAILBLAZING

PART V:
MIND MATTERS

PART VI:
BEAUTY BASICS

INTRODUCTION

Breakthrough! The word conjures up images of arms raised in triumph, faces lit up with smiles, and eyes lifted up to the sky. It's cause for celebration! And this book is filled with them—hundreds of breakthroughs in both health and weight loss gathered together to help you to improve your health, your size, and your life.

Part I: Health Breakthroughs offers the latest information on wellness. You'll read all about the remarkable innovations in detection and treatment that will dramatically impact your health—and the health of the people you love. You'll discover strategies based on the latest and best scientific research to nurture four essential systems and keep you fabulous for a lifetime. Find eight natural remedies to relieve your pain—fast. And learn the nine simple changes to make to your life that can add up to better health.

In Part II: Nutrition News you'll learn how to improve your diet just by making some simple substitutions. Then taste the new generation of health-boosting foods that do double or triple duty to help prevent illness. (There's broccoli or fungi among them!) Discover how to beat fatigue by eating the right foods and stay energized, sharp, and focused all day. Plus, learn how to go organic—without spending a ton of green.

The latest and greatest weight-loss breakthroughs are center stage in Part III: Weight-Loss Wisdom. Learn why it might be time to say "Welcome back, carbs." Discover the right way to lose fat at 40 plus. Find out the secret to never overeat again. And make a few small adjustments in your life to finally, finally lose those last 10 pounds for good.

Get a move on in Part IV: Fitness Trailblazing. You'll see how to get your fitness "party" started on the right foot. Walk off five times more weight with our fastest-ever routine. Discover how small movements you can add to your life can add up to big-time fitness and weight loss. You'll never think about tapping a pencil the same way again.

In Part V: Mind Matters is where you'll read all about your mental health. Let your brain reign and do everything a little quicker, easier, and better. Start every day off right with our simple three-step plan. Yep, it's gonna be a great day! Tap into your bright side and reap the benefits that truly happy people enjoy.

Part VI: Beauty Basics will help you to look great, for life. Give Father Time a little kick in the pants with our breakthrough treatments and insider secrets. Learn how to supplement your skin care and get beautiful from the inside out. Defy your age with the top doctor-recommended products that are only as far away as your corner drugstore. And finally, peer into a beautiful future with the most cutting-edge innovations that will make you look as young as you feel.

We hope that this book filled with breakthroughs will help you to have some major breakthroughs of your own. Here's to your health and happiness!

PART

HEALTH
BREAKTHROUGHS

ARM YOURSELF WITH INFORMATION

Remarkable innovations in detection and treatment are making a stunning impact on health

They don't call it the "information age" for nothing. These days knowledge is power. The more you know today, the better off you'll be tomorrow.

Over the past 12 months, cutting-edge scientists have unveiled an astonishing array of drugs, devices, and treatments that foreshadow a fresh approach to preventing and conquering disease. With the help of our esteemed editorial advisors, we assembled a list of the most impressive among them, then asked ourselves which advances would most interest our readers and their families. From noninvasive alternatives to breast biopsies to new weapons against deadly infections, here are the most promising health advances of the past year.

BREAKTHROUGH THAT
COULD WIPE OUT "SUPERBUGS"

Researchers at the University of North Carolina at Chapel Hill discovered a new weapon to fight the growing threat of drug-resistant bacteria, and it may already be in your medicine cabinet. Bisphosphonates—compounds in the bone-building drug Didronel—prevent superbugs from sharing their DNA, halting the spread of resistant strains.

"Even more surprising, bisphosphonates kill cells that harbor resistant DNA, selectively eliminating the most dangerous germs," says Matt Redinbo, PhD, a professor of chemistry, biochemistry, and biophysics at the university. Some doctors are already prescribing bisphosphonates off-label to fight infections, though the drugs can have side effects such as gastrointestinal irritation and bone damage in the jaw.

BREAKTHROUGH THAT SPEEDS
TREATMENT OF VAGINAL INFECTIONS

Probiotics—friendly bacteria that thrive in the body—are known to prevent or even cure yeast infections and bacterial vaginosis. Now there's an over-the-counter supplement containing the two Lactobacillus strains documented to promote vaginal health.

The probiotic pill Fem-Dophilus has erased up to 90 percent of vaginal bacterial infections and significantly reduced yeast growth in trials by coating the lining of vaginal tissues and producing acids that keep pathogens from gaining a foothold. And when women take antibiotics, Fem-Dophilus doubles the drugs' effectiveness by recolonizing the vagina with healthy flora.

BREAKTHROUGH THAT RESTORES
NECK MOVEMENT AFTER SURGERY

People with cervical degenerative disk disease who receive a new flexible artificial disk implant can bend their necks normally after surgery—a vast improvement over people who undergo standard spinal fusion, a procedure in which a surgeon removes the diseased disk and locks adjoining vertebrae, limiting range of motion.

In a 2-year, 541-patient clinical trial, people who received the Prestige Cervical Disc System from Medtronic (approved by the FDA in July) had greater range of motion, felt less pain, and returned to work 16 days faster than those who got the standard treatment. A 7-year follow-up study is under way to evaluate long-term safety and effectiveness.

BREAKTHROUGH THAT COULD PREVENT 90 PERCENT OF OVARIAN CANCER DEATHS

Ovarian cancer, a stealthy killer responsible for about 15,000 deaths in 2007, may not be so silent after all: Recent studies show that even early-stage ovarian cancer reveals itself with subtle symptoms up to a year before typical diagnosis. (See "Recurring Symptoms Women Shouldn't Ignore" below.)

Now the American Cancer Society is spreading the word. When cancer is detected while it's still confined to the ovary, you have a 90 percent

RECURRING SYMPTOMS
WOMEN SHOULDN'T IGNORE

See a gynecologist ASAP if you have the following symptoms almost daily and they last more than a few weeks.

- Pelvic or abdominal pain
- Bloating
- Feeling full quickly or having difficulty eating
- Having to urinate often or feeling an urgent need to go

COMING SOON

Our experts rave about these in-the-works innovations.

A WAY TO HEAL THE HEART WITHOUT BYPASS SURGERY: Using an injected drug that spurs blood vessel growth, researchers in Germany have boosted heart patients' performance in exercise tests by 80 percent while reducing symptoms such as angina and chest pain. Animal studies in the United States by the biotech company CardioVascular BioTherapeutics suggest the drug's active ingredient, fibroblast growth factor, also reduces brain damage from stroke. The drug has passed US safety tests and is green-lighted by the FDA for clinical trials for severe coronary disease.

A VACCINE FOR MS: The first vaccine for autoimmune diseases may help combat multiple sclerosis, type 1 diabetes, lupus, rheumatoid arthritis, and other immune system diseases that collectively affect up to 24 million people. Results published in the *Archives of Neurology* show that the vaccine limits production of activated immune cells called T cells, which cause the chronic inflammation characteristic of MS. It's now headed for more clinical trials.

A DRUG THAT FIGHTS ALZHEIMER'S DISEASE: The first Alzheimer's drug that blocks the disease rather than just fighting symptoms has passed efficacy trials at six sites around the country. The once-a-day pill is a compound known as a gamma-secretase inhibitor, which interferes with an enzyme that produces the brain-clogging plaques that characterize Alzheimer's, reducing them by 38 percent, according to preliminary results.

A MOLECULE THAT MAKES CANCER SELF-DESTRUCT: Canadian researchers believe they've developed a simple molecule that dramatically slows tumor growth without affecting healthy cells. Called DCA (dichloroacetate), the novel compound revives mitochondria—power packets in cells that regulate cell death but are switched off by cancer. By flipping the "on" switch of an enzyme, DCA commands abnormal cells to destroy cancer from within.

chance of being cured, but those odds drop to 20 percent if the cancer is advanced, which is when it's usually diagnosed. Telltale symptoms are common and often due to something other than cancer, so you don't have to worry about every bloating episode. But if symptoms occur almost daily and last more than a few weeks, the American Cancer Society recommends seeing a gynecologist.

BREAKTHROUGH THAT COULD SAVE MILLIONS OF LIVES

If you're not revived within 5 minutes after cardiac arrest, you're as good as dead. But researchers now know that the window of time for survival could triple if the body is cooled by several degrees soon after the heart stops beating. In hospitals, doctors are using cooling blankets that circulate icy water to minimize brain damage and revive "temporarily dead" people who had no heartbeat for up to 15 minutes, according to Lance Becker, MD, director of the Center for Resuscitation Science at the University of Pennsylvania.

In a 2007 animal study, cooling boosted the rate of survival immediately after cardiac arrest from 10 to 60 percent, Dr. Becker says. Researchers are now trying to develop an injectable, icy slurry that lowers body temperature within seconds and that emergency workers could administer on the spot. (Doctors say putting ice or cold compresses on a heart attack victim at home is unlikely to help much: The brain and organs are too well insulated to be affected by simple aids.)

BREAKTHROUGH THAT TAKES THE FEAR— AND WAITING—OUT OF BREAST BIOPSIES

A new ultrasound technique called elasticity imaging can determine with nearly 100 percent accuracy whether breast lesions are cancerous or harmless without a surgical sample. The FDA-approved system combines a manual exam with scanning to gauge how tissue inside the breast moves when pushed; malignant growths appear stiffer.

Developers say elasticity imaging could reduce unnecessary breast procedures—80 percent of breast biopsies turn out to be benign, according to the American Cancer Society—and spare women days of anxiety waiting for biopsy results. "Decreasing invasiveness while increasing accuracy and convenience makes this a great technology," says *Prevention* advisor Pamela Peeke, MD, an assistant professor of medicine at the University of Maryland School of Medicine.

BREAKTHROUGH THAT REDUCES MENOPAUSE SYMPTOMS BY HALF

A fast-drying, colorless gel absorbed by the skin, Elestrin treats moderate to severe hot flashes by delivering an effective low estrogen dose (0.0125 milligram). That's important: The American College of Obstetricians and Gynecologists recommends using the lowest effective dose of estrogen for the shortest time because of possible cardiovascular and cancer risks.

Four to 5 weeks into clinical trials, women using Elestrin had fewer and less severe hot flashes—usually reducing symptoms by half or more—followed by greater relief each week for most of the 12-week study.

BREAKTHROUGH THAT COULD WARN OF DIABETES YEARS BEFORE IT DEVELOPS

Tests for three proteins—all telltale signs of inflammation that are linked to insulin resistance—can predict whether women will develop diabetes years before standard screenings indicate a problem. In a 6-year study of more than 82,000 women ages 50 and older, researchers at UCLA found that the tests (already available but not widely used) accurately warned of diabetes even in people with normal blood sugar. Early alerts could enable those at high risk to make preemptive lifestyle changes and potentially help prevent the disease.

BREAKTHROUGH THAT MAKES MAMMOGRAMS MORE ACCURATE AND COMFORTABLE

A low-radiation three-dimensional mammography CT developed at Duke University is twice as accurate and much less painful than scans that flatten the breast. Women lie facedown on a bed with a cutout for the breast while the scanner circles it from below, eliminating distortion found in standard images of compressed breasts. However, developers say commercial use is still years away.

BEST UPGRADES

The following four proven tools are getting even better.

AN EFFECTIVE FAUX ARTERY: Synthetic grafts used in bypass operations are now more successful with the Gore Propaten Vascular Graft, which bonds the anticoagulant drug heparin to the surface of an artificial blood vessel. The embedded drug prevents blood clots formed in response to grafts created with veins or other synthetic blood vessels.

AN INSULIN PEN WITH A MEMORY: People with diabetes can keep better track of insulin injections with the first digital pen dispenser that records time and dosage data. The memory capability of HumaPen Memoir should mean better blood sugar control for forgetful patients.

CATHETERS THAT CONQUER INFECTION: A new antimicrobial silver coating for bacteria-prone medical devices, such as catheters, is impervious to bacteria that cause 99,000 infection deaths in US hospitals a year. Nanotechnology that's used to treat tube surfaces can keep them antiseptic for months at a time.

A QUICKER, SAFER CT SCAN: CT scans of the heart using the GE LightSpeed VCT XT expose patients to 70 percent less radiation than conventional CT scans by taking images in rapid-fire sequence rather than in one continuous exposure. Scans are completed in as little as 5 seconds instead of the 10- to 12-second exposures needed with older CT machines.

BREAKTHROUGH THAT COULD HELP STROKE VICTIMS WALK AGAIN

Stroke and other neurological impairments often cause "foot drop"—a gait condition in which patients can't step heel first, making it difficult to walk without stumbling. A new system called the NESS L300 uses a sensor in the shoe to tell a lightweight wireless device worn below the knee when the heel is on or off the ground. With this information, the device sends electrical pulses to the leg nerve that controls lifting the foot so that some patients can walk more naturally.

"This is a huge improvement over wearing a brace," says Gad Alon, PhD, PT, an associate professor in the department of physical therapy and rehabilitation science at the University of Maryland School of Medicine.

BREAKTHROUGH THAT PROTECTS BONES IN ONE 15-MINUTE DOSE

Half of people on oral bone-building drugs don't keep up with their meds, probably because irritating side effects, such as stomach pain, are common. They take less than 80 percent of their prescribed pills each year.

That's not an issue with Reclast, a new medication for treating postmenopausal osteoporosis that's given just once annually in a 15-minute infusion. Reclast improved bone density, reducing spine fractures by 70 percent and hip fractures by 41 percent, compared with a placebo, in a 3-year clinical trial of 7,765 women. Administering the infusion directly into the bloodstream eliminates digestive problems that are common with oral meds; Reclast's side effects, such as fever and bone or muscle pain, usually disappear within 3 days.

fast fact
60: Number of countries Diane M. Harper visited (see next page) in a single year on her mission against cervical cancer

HEALTH HEROES

She helped develop a vaccine that could save 250,000 women a year

Her mother died young of cancer—and Diane M. Harper, MD, MPH, has been fighting the disease ever since. A researcher, clinician, and professor at Dartmouth Medical School, Harper, 50, helped design and run studies that led to the approval of the first vaccine against human papillomavirus, the main cause of cervical cancer. Now she's crisscrossing the globe to educate doctors on how best to use it. "A woman dies of cervical cancer every 2 minutes," she says. "This can save lives."

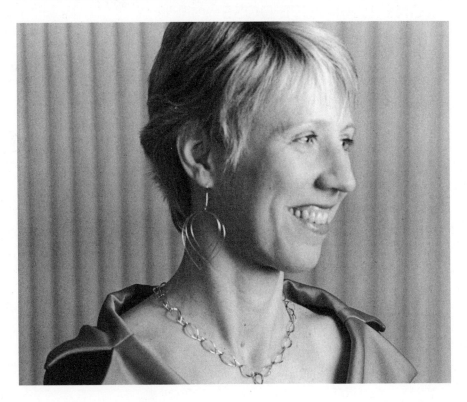

STOP THE CLOCK!

Longevity researchers are discovering why some people resist age-related diseases and live a century or longer

There's no avoiding it: Aging is inevitable, and it's happening now. Longevity experts are tackling the issue of aging at unprecedented rates, and they're making breakthroughs in extending the life of many creatures, from a simple yeast cell to more complex animals such as mice and monkeys. History tells us that as medical advances continue to evolve, the average life span of people will increase. In the year 2000, there were only about 72,000 centenarians, or people who are at least 100 years old, in America. According to the US Census Bureau, when the year 2050 rolls around, about 834,000 Americans will be at least 100 years old. That's a group larger than the population of San Francisco!

In laboratories around the world, researchers are peeking into our very cells to determine what kinds of changes occur over time, and almost all of them agree: We can control the rate at which we age. There's no denying that genetics play a role in determining life span, but lifestyle plays an even greater part. One Swedish study on twins who were raised in the same household versus different ones (thus being influenced by the same genes but perhaps different environments) estimated that longevity differences are about 35 percent genetic and 65 percent environmental. Other studies on twins have found that inherited factors account for only 25 to 30 percent of longevity.

Although you can't go back and pick different parents, you can pick the foods you eat, the exercise plans you follow, and whether or not you smoke. All of these decisions go a long way toward determining whether or not you'll live to a healthy ripe age.

There are hundreds of ways to slow down or even prevent the conditions that are responsible for many deaths and disabilities in later years. Here are strategies based on the latest and best scientific research to nurture four essential systems and keep you fabulous for a lifetime.

THE CARDIOVASCULAR SYSTEM

Your goal: Prevent a heart attack

How You Age

Cholesterol levels shift. HDL (good) cholesterol sweeps up LDL (bad) cholesterol and shunts it to the liver for removal. As you age, the levels of HDL can drop off, so the bad stuff builds up, causing plaque.

Plaque causes clots. Plaque burrows into and inflames artery walls. When a plaque deposit bursts, the body's healing mechanism produces a clot, which can cause a heart attack.

Arteries become weak and stiff. High blood pressure hardens flexible arteries, which strains the heart, rips open plaque deposits, and promotes blood vessel leaks that can cause an aneurysm or a stroke.

Blood can become "sticky." High blood sugar is like a soda spill on a countertop; it permits plaque-forming material to fasten more easily to artery walls. It's also a symptom of diabetes, which doubles your risk of heart disease or stroke.

Waist size expands. Slowing metabolism leads to weight gain, which contributes to diabetes, high blood pressure, and high cholesterol. "Large waist size is the most important risk factor; it compounds all the others," says Annabelle Volgman, MD, medical director of the Heart Center for Women at Rush University Medical Center in Chicago.

Your Stay-Young Plan

Keep moving. "Physical activity reduces every controllable risk factor," says Dr. Volgman. Just 10 minutes of cardiovascular exercise on most days can cut a sedentary person's heart attack risk in half. By boosting aerobic fitness and metabolism, twice-a-week interval training (short bursts of high-intensity exercise) for just 2 weeks can reduce heart risks by 20 percent, according to studies. To get started, simply vary the pace of your daily walk for 2 minutes every 10.

Eat more omega-3 fatty acids. They curb inflammation, lower blood pressure, and slow plaque growth. To get more, eat oily fish such as salmon at least twice a week and consider taking fish oil (EPA and DHA) supplements of 850 to 1,000 milligrams a day if you have heart disease.

Take an aspirin with a doctor's okay. Low doses prevent clots that cause heart attacks, but regular use can cause stomach bleeding and increased stroke risk. "Whether you should take it depends on your age and family history," says Lori Mosca, MD, PhD, an associate professor of medicine at Columbia University in New York City.

Load up on antioxidants. Stock your shelves like the Mediterraneans, with olive oil, leafy greens, whole grains, nuts, fish, red wine, and tomatoes. Their rich blend of antioxidants, phytochemicals, vitamins, and healthy fats cuts cardiovascular risks. Just 3 months of Mediterranean-style eating in one study improved blood sugar, blood pressure, and cholesterol in people at high risk of heart disease.

Avoid antioxidant supplements. Recent research suggests that high doses of beta-carotene, vitamin A, and vitamin E may increase the risk of premature death, and too much vitamin C may boost the risk of dying for women over the age of 50 with diabetes.

Cut saturated fat even further. Artery-damaging fat should account for less than 10 percent of daily calories. Ideally, you should keep it below 7 percent. Be vigilant about reading food labels to avoid eating partially hydrogenated (trans) fats.

Trim 200 calories a day after menopause. After 50, women's metabolism slows about 5 percent a decade, so the body burns less energy.

Monitor your markers. Keep a copy of the blood work you have done during your annual physical and track changes over time. Make sure your numbers are always within the following ranges.

- Cholesterol: LDL under 100 mg/dL; HDL above 50
- Blood pressure: Below 120/80 mm Hg
- Fasting blood sugar: Less than 100 mg/dL
- Triglycerides: Less than 150 mg/dL

If you have heart disease or are at risk for it, ask for a test called lipo-protein subfraction, which measures the size of your cholesterol particles. If your LDL particles are very small, they are better able to burrow into artery walls, despite normal or low cholesterol readings, so you may need more aggressive monitoring and treatment.

Test for inflammation. Doctors know that when LDL cholesterol damages the arterial wall, the artery becomes chronically inflamed, starting a cascade of events that may culminate in a heart attack. As part of this inflammatory response, your body produces a substance called C-reactive protein (CRP), which can be measured in a blood test. If you have normal cholesterol but a high level of CRP, you may need a more aggressive preventive plan (more intense monitoring of lipids).

Brush your teeth; clean your arteries. Cutting your risk of heart disease may be as easy as regularly flossing and brushing. Columbia Uni-

fast fact --
In the average lifetime, the heart beats 2.5 billion times.
----

versity doctors have found that people whose mouths contain a high number of the bacteria that cause gum disease are more likely to have plaque-clogged arteries. Pay particular attention to receding gums. A study found that men ages 40 to 75 who had lost eight or more teeth because of gum disease had a 57 percent higher risk of stroke than those who had lost fewer than eight.

Get a baseline heart scan. Prominent cardiologists recommend that women over age 50 who are postmenopausal and have any risk factors for coronary disease get a heart scan—several different technologies are available—to measure coronary artery calcium, which directly correlates to the total amount of plaque in your arteries. An early baseline enables your doctor to monitor signs of heart disease. One of the best technologies is the 64-slice CT scanner, which measures calcium and the amount of dangerous soft plaque in the arteries. Filled primarily with cholesterol, soft plaque is prone to rupture, resulting in a blood clot that can cause a heart attack.

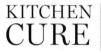

KITCHEN CURE | Eating a 30-calorie square of dark chocolate daily for 2 weeks will lower systolic blood pressure by 3 points and diastolic pressure by 2.

THE BRAIN

Your goal: Stay sharp

How You Age

Your gray matter shrinks. Neurons start diminishing in number and size, slightly reducing brain volume and your ability to recall details and facts with the quickness of your youth.

Tangles and plaques destroy cells. Tangles are fibers that develop inside neurons; plaques are a buildup of sticky proteins between neurons—both are thought to knot up and kill nerve cells. Having some tangles and plaques is normal, but developing too many is associated with Alzheimer's disease.

Free radical damage accumulates. Inside brain cells, free radicals can damage DNA and interfere with energy-producing mitochondria, causing premature cell death.

Connections between neurons diminish. Levels of a neurotransmitter directly involved in memory, called acetylcholine, naturally decrease with age, reducing the brain's ability to transport messages from one cell to another.

Stress takes a toll. Long periods of anxiety and worry may harm your brain, especially the hippocampus—responsible for memory. A Rush University Medical Center study followed more than 1,200 people over 12 years and found those most easily stressed developed more cognitive impairment by the end of the study than other participants did.

High blood pressure and cholesterol starve cells. LDL cholesterol can clog tiny capillaries in the brain, cutting off the blood that supplies oxygen, nutrients, and energizing glucose and increasing the risk of stroke. High blood pressure doubles your risk of Alzheimer's.

Your Stay-Young Plan

Give your brain some quiet time. Adequate sleep makes you smarter. Research from the sleep disorders program at Massachusetts General Hospital in Boston shows that sleep helps the brain bring together disparate pieces of information and interpret them correctly. Conversely, too little sleep leads to bad performance and mood disorders. Another way to refresh the brain is meditation. Regular meditators' brains exhibit high levels of gamma waves, associated with attention, working memory, and learning. Emory University researchers also discovered that when people

fast fact
66: The percentage reduction in stress hormone levels in women who meditate, compared with nonmeditators

begin meditating in middle age, they experience less loss of gray matter and attention levels when compared with those who do not meditate.

Go fish. Omega-3 fatty acids are especially beneficial. Found in fish such as salmon, halibut, and sardines, these fatty acids are involved in nerve cell communication. Research shows they help protect against the cell damage that leads to Alzheimer's. Consider getting your omega-3s in pill form. Unlike whole fish, supplements have been found to be free of mercury and PCBs, according to analyses by ConsumerLab.com.

Embrace fitness. Exercise produces large quantities of brain-derived neurotrophic factor (BDNF), which is a protein that helps neurons survive and encourages the growth of new ones. "I call it Miracle-Gro for the brain," says John Ratey, MD, a clinical associate professor of psychiatry at Harvard Medical School and author of *Spark: The Revolutionary New Science of Exercise and the Brain.* "It helps the cells grow and makes them better and more resilient to future stresses." Brains with more BDNF have a greater capacity for knowledge. To boost BDNF levels, Dr. Ratey recommends moderate- to high-intensity aerobic exercise, incorporating interval training. Other research shows that just walking brings substantial benefits. Best bet: Include a 10-minute speedwalk in your daily stroll.

When you add strength training to your routine, you'll boost your brain even more. The latest research shows that muscle-building activities such as yoga and lightweight workouts increase production of IGF-1, which is another chemical essential to the growth of neurons.

Seek novelty. Your brain is a thrill seeker. New experiences stimulate the area that produces dopamine, which is a chemical involved in learning and memory. It also loves a brand-new workout. Studies show that doing new things builds brain mass and increases mental agility. The absence of novelty, however, causes dopamine-producing areas of the brain to shrink. To keep your brain lithe and strong, take up a language, hobby, sport, or musical instrument—any regular pastime that offers continual fresh challenge. Even if you're not good at your new pursuit, you'll still get the benefits.

Stay connected. The brain grows—even in old age—in response to pats, hugs, and other physical affection. Regular socializing also keeps your brain sharp by reducing cortisol, the destructive stress hormone. When scientists at Rush University performed postmortems on the brains of 89 seniors, they were surprised to find plaques and tangles associated with Alzheimer's in several of the deceased, though none had experienced any of the disease's telltale symptoms. When they researched the seniors' social histories, they found the deceased all had one thing in common: tight relationships with many friends and family members.

Dancing is a great way to strengthen connections, both socially and neurologically. In a study from McGill University in Canada, seniors 62 and older who tangoed for 4 hours a week for 10 weeks improved their memories. Don't like dancing? Go shopping at the mall with a friend, which offers the same benefits. When you're shopping, you're socializing, figuring out the best bargains, and walking without even realizing you're getting in a workout.

KITCHEN CURE

Apples truly do keep the doctor away. They contain antioxidants that raise levels of acetylcholine, a neurotransmitter directly involved in memory. Apples also contain quercetin, which is a flavonoid that protects brain cells against damage from free radicals.

BONES AND JOINTS

Your goal: Be active for life

How You Age

Bones get thin. After bone mass peaks around age 30, you start to lose 1 to 2 percent of bone a year. That pace accelerates quickly for women, who lose 3 or 4 percent annually in the first 5 to 7 years after menopause, when declining estrogen offers less protection against cells called osteoclasts that break down bone. This puts you at high risk of both osteoporosis and fractures, its most serious consequences. By the age of 65 or 70, men and women lose bone density at the same rate, so both sexes are at risk for fractures.

Muscle fibers shorten and weaken. Around age 40, muscles start shrinking and losing energy-producing mitochondria in their cells. Weakened, poorly nourished muscles have lower aerobic capacity and absorb sugar from the bloodstream less efficiently, making bone-building exercise difficult.

Joints lose their cushions. Synovial fluid, which lubricates the protective cartilage in knee, hip, and other joints, begins to dry. Cartilage then erodes and frays, a precursor to arthritis.

Interestingly, about 26 percent of women get arthritis, compared with only 17 percent of men. Experts believe the reason why is that muscles attached to wider pelvises exert additional stress on knees that, over time, exacerbates cartilage damage.

Your Stay-Young Plan

Do weight-bearing exercise. Walking, dancing, stairclimbing, skiing—any activity that forces your skeleton to support your weight—speeds the work of bone-building osteoblast cells. Just a half hour of brisk walking boosted two measures of bone growth in one study. But avoid high-impact moves such as running or jumping if you already have osteoporosis or are at risk for fractures.

When deciding which activity suits you best, consider tai chi. Postmenopausal women who've practiced the slow, graceful movements of this exercise for years have denser bones, and even beginners slow bone loss as soon as they start tai chi programs, according to a research review at Harvard University.

Strengthen and tone your muscles. The stronger you are, the less likely you'll be injured in a fall. What's more, lifting weights as little as twice a week reverses loss of mitochondria, giving you and your muscles extra energy, according to a study at the Buck Institute for Age Research in Novato, California. A 16-week strength-training program has also been shown to cut arthritis pain by 43 percent. Bonus benefit: Muscle workouts boost your metabolic rate by as much as 15 percent, so you burn more calories even when you're inactive.

People with strong thighs have less cartilage damage and pain in their knees from osteoarthritis, according to one study, so be sure to target your quadriceps. Mayo Clinic researchers say toned quads reduce lateral kneecap motion that speeds cartilage wear. Be sure also to strengthen your hamstrings at the backs of your thighs so you don't create muscle imbalance.

Get enough calcium. The mineral is the main component of bone, and men and women need at least 1,000 milligrams a day. Women should increase this dose to 1,200 milligrams after menopause, and men should match that intake when they turn 51. Yet 78 percent of us don't get enough, especially after age 50, when adult intake averages just 674 milligrams a day. Eat calcium-rich dairy foods and consider taking two 500-milligram supplements a day.

"Take doses separately—for example, one at breakfast and one at dinner," says Kimberly Templeton, MD, an associate professor of orthopedic surgery at the University of Kansas Medical Center in Kansas City. "The body can absorb only about 500 milligrams at a time."

Additional food sources include fat-free milk, 1 cup of which provides one-third of the Daily Value for calcium, and spinach, which delivers 12 percent of the DV for calcium and also contains vitamin C, a collagen builder that improves calcium absorption.

You should also supplement your diet with vitamin D. It helps calcium enter the bloodstream and fuse to bone, but half of women aren't getting the 200 IU recommended before menopause—much less the 400 IU that all of us should get after age 50. What's more, many experts think that the current recommendation is too low, prompting the National Osteoporosis Foundation to raise its recommendation to 800 to 1,000 IU of D a day for adults 50 and older.

Here's a fast food fix: 3.5 ounces of salmon provides 90 percent of the DV for vitamin D, contains bone-building calcium, and is rich in omega-3 fatty acids, which reduce inflammation linked to rheumatoid arthritis.

Stay ahead of arthritis pain with massage and acupuncture. These two natural treatments are known to ease pain, with none of the potentially serious gastrointestinal side effects caused by nonsteroidal anti-inflammatory drugs (also known as NSAIDs) such as ibuprofen. Studies have shown that stimulation of pressure points, either manually or with acupuncture needles, prompts the nervous system to release chemicals that mask pain.

Have a bone scan, when the time is right. Bones don't let on that they're weak—until they break. That's why you should get a bone mineral density test such as a dual-energy x-ray absorptiometry (DEXA) if you meet the following criteria from the National Osteoporosis Foundation.

Women: You're postmenopausal and under the age of 65, have a fractured bone, or have any risk factor for osteoporosis—you are thin, are small-framed, exercise very little, don't get enough calcium and vitamin D, smoke cigarettes, or have recently quit smoking after many years. Without risk factors, you should have the test if you're 65 or older.

Men: You're between 50 and 70 years old, have a fractured bone, have any risk factors for osteoporosis, experience sudden back pain, or notice changes in your height and posture. Without risk factors, you should have the test if you're 70 or older.

KITCHEN CURE

For a delicious way to ease arthritis pain, drink pomegranate juice. In lab tests done at Case Western Reserve University and reported in the *Journal of Nutrition*, extract from the fruit lowered levels of an inflammatory chemical called interleukin-1B, which is released during arthritis flare-ups, as well as enzymes that erode cartilage.

SKIN

Your goal: Look younger

How You Age

Cell turnover slows. Through the natural exfoliation process, your skin sheds dead cells as younger ones, generated deep in the epidermis (skin's top layer), migrate upward to replace them. In young, healthy skin, cells take about 28 days to reach the surface and flake off 12 days later. As you age, renewal slows: New cells aren't produced as quickly, and old ones hang on longer.

Free radicals attack. The body is assaulted by unstable oxygen molecules—called free radicals—from pollution, stress, cigarette smoke, and the skin's top enemy, the sun. Over many years, this causes cell irregularities, including discoloration and cancer.

Collagen breaks down. After age 40, the body typically slows down the rate at which it produces collagen, which is a mesh of protein that, together with elastin, helps keep your skin plump and elastic. When collagen degrades and is not replaced at the same rate, the outer skin loses volume and settles into creases and wrinkles.

Skin dries out. Your cells lose moisture faster after age 40, as estrogen production and thyroid function—both of which affect sweat glands—slow down.

Your Stay-Young Plan

Cover up. Avoid the sun as much as possible. Stay in the shade between 10 a.m. and 2 p.m., when UV rays are strongest, and wear a wide-brimmed hat and clothing that covers much of your body. Apply sunscreen every morning—a shot glass–full, slathered on thick.

Dermatologists have changed their sunblock recommendations for extended sun exposure from a sun protection factor (SPF) of 15, which blocks 93 percent of the sun's radiation, to a broad-spectrum SPF 30, which blocks 97 percent and protects against both UVB rays (which typically cause sunburn) and UVAs (which age the skin more gradually).

For skin that's already faced years of sun exposure, that extra 4 percent can make a big difference in preventing further damage. Your SPF 15 products are still okay to wear if you spend most of your days indoors and get little exposure to the sun.

Get adequate sleep. They don't call it *beauty sleep* for nothing. Skin cells regenerate more quickly when you snooze. Dark circles under the eyes are the immediate consequence of losing just a few hours of restorative sleep. Prolonged sleep deprivation can lead to dry, dull skin all over the body.

Before you snooze, apply moisturizer. The temperature of your skin rises slightly when you're asleep, helping it absorb creams and lotions. Antiaging potions may also work better because they're not competing with makeup or sun exposure. Try a bedtime-specific cream such as ROC Retinol Correxion Deep Wrinkle Night Cream; evening formulas are often richer than daytime formulas but don't contain SPF. Slather dry feet, hands, and nails with a rich, hydrating cream or petroleum jelly.

Drink more water. Downing six to eight glasses of water each day helps skin stay elastic and supple, says Doris J. Day, MD, a clinical assistant professor of dermatology at New York University Medical Center. "When the skin is adequately hydrated, it looks healthier and more vibrant, and makes some wrinkles less visible."

Destress. Stress—both internal and external—makes the body's defense mechanisms work overtime and deprives skin of moisture, leaving it drier and more vulnerable to irritants and allergens. Unwind during the day with quick periods of meditation or focused breathing—and do a quick exercise DVD (kickboxing?) after work. Just be sure to pick a mindful activity during which you are tuned in to your body and not distracted by your blasting iPod.

Do cardio. "Think of the flush on your face after a good workout: That's a sign that your skin's getting the oxygen and nutrients it needs," says Audrey Kunin, MD, a Kansas City, Missouri–based dermatologist and author of *The DERMAdoctor Skinstruction Manual*. A good sweat flushes impurities from pores while you're burning calories and keeping off extra pounds that could put unnecessary strain on the skin. Before you work out, make sure you're well hydrated and use extra moisturizer, particularly in the drier, colder months.

Try yoga. "Stretching tones and conditions the muscles and firms up the skin they're attached to," says Hema Sundaram, MD, a Washington, DC–area dermatologist and cosmetic surgeon. Backward-bending poses such as the fish, camel, and cobra can counter gravity's pull when done regularly, while the forward-bending child, bowing sun salutation, and headstand poses encourage a rich supply of blood to the face. And the more you can truly relax your facial muscles, the less you're contributing to future crow's-feet, frown lines, and wrinkles.

Eat antioxidants. If skin's biggest enemies are free radicals, its best friends are the vitamins and minerals that neutralize the volatile and destructive molecules. Eating lots of antioxidants—five to eight servings of fruits and vegetables a day—can combat cellular damage caused by free radicals.

KITCHEN CURE

For a simple antioxidant brew to battle free radicals and fight cellular damage, boil water, add a green tea bag, and sip. People who do so regularly have less sun-related skin damage than those who don't, according to Dartmouth Medical School researchers. The tonic, which contains the powerful antioxidant EGCG, can be used as a topical ingredient as well. Ask your dermatologist about Replenix, available in doctor's offices.

DECODE YOUR ZIP CODE

The quality of health care across the United States varies to an alarming degree

For weeks you've suffered from yet another bout of back pain so severe you can hardly get out of bed in the morning. Your family doctor and the orthopedic surgeon she referred you to both say you're a good candidate for spine surgery. And it seems like everyone is having it—your next-door neighbor, your boss, the waitress at your favorite restaurant. You set a date for the procedure.

But what if you knew that your town had one of the highest rates of back surgery in the United States, nearly three times the national average? And that an orthopedic surgeon 50 miles away would advise you to wait a while and see whether the pain went away on its own? Would that change your decision?

Mounting research suggests that where you live plays a significant role in the health care you receive. "We've found that geography is often destiny," says James N. Weinstein, DO, MPH, director of the Dartmouth Institute for Health Policy and Clinical Practice, where this field of study was pioneered. "It's not that the rates of disease are different, it's the way they're treated that's different—from prevention to diagnosis to long-term care."

Luckily, you don't have to accept the health care your neighborhood allots you. By asking pointed questions of your physician, for instance, or knowing when to seek a second opinion from a specialist in another state, you can turn these differences to your advantage. (See "Four Keys to Great Health Care.") Here are the region-by-region facts, as well as local hot spots that have questionable (or progressive) practices, and—most important—expert advice on how to use this information to get the very best health care, wherever you call home.

THE WEST

The states: Alaska, Arizona, California, Colorado, Hawaii, Idaho, Montana, Nevada, New Mexico, Oregon, Utah, Washington, and Wyoming

Prevention is neglected. When it comes to women's preventive health care, the West scores low. In 2006, less than 70 percent of women over age 40 in "big sky" states such as Idaho, Utah, and Wyoming had gotten a mammogram in the past 2 years, compared with the national average of 77 percent, according to the Centers for Disease Control and Prevention (CDC). The proportion of women getting Pap tests is also relatively low—though both tests have been shown to save lives by detecting cancer in treatable stages. Another preventive tool, cholesterol screening, also lags in many of these states.

Patients are informed. Medical decisions aren't always clear-cut. One person with terminal cancer, for instance, might want to try all available options, no matter how grueling, while another might prefer to enjoy her remaining days free of treatment and its side effects. In other words, the "right" decision is often a matter of how a person weighs the pros and cons. With a pilot project started in 2007, Washington became the first state to push doctors to share all relevant information with anyone facing an important elective surgery. Experts say that those discussions are critical in allowing the patient's values to guide the decision.

FOUR KEYS TO GREAT HEALTH CARE

Although you may not have much control over the quality of health care in your area, you can do many things to receive the treatment you deserve in the doctor's office. Here are four powerful prescriptions for successful medical care.

FIND A DOCTOR YOU TRUST—AND WHO LISTENS. If your physician treats you like a customer at a drive-thru or makes you feel foolish for asking questions, get another doctor. Experts say protect yourself and find a physician who will explain a procedure's risks and benefits and listen to your personal concerns.

EXPLORE THE DO-NOTHING OPTION. "If a doctor recommends an invasive treatment, such as a hysterectomy or knee surgery, you should ask a series of questions," advises Shannon Brownlee, author of *Overtreated: Why Too Much Medicine Is Making Us Sicker and Poorer*. "Ask: Is there a less invasive treatment I can try first? What's the evidence this treatment will leave me better off than I am now? How good is the evidence? What's likely to happen if I don't do anything?"

Query tests, too. Experts know tests can reveal an abnormality that may never cause a problem, but once a little abnormality is found, it's hard for a doctor (or a patient) to do nothing.

FIND A SECOND OPINION OUTSIDE YOUR COMMUNITY. If your condition is serious (or can be treated multiple ways), it's worth traveling across town to a doctor affiliated with a different hospital—or perhaps even to another state to see a doctor there. Or get another point of view without hitting the road by trying a reputable online service that offers second opinions, such as MyConsult, run by the Cleveland Clinic. Visit www.eclevelandclinic.org/myConsultHome and search on "MyConsult." Bear in mind that the cost of online second opinions may not be covered by your insurance.

SEEK DECISION-MAKING TOOLS. Many medical choices have no obvious right or wrong answer, only ones that work better or worse for you. In the case of breast cancer, for instance, one woman might prefer to preserve her breast—even though she'll have to be alert to the possibility of the tumor recurring—while another woman might choose to have a mastectomy. At decisionaid.ohri.ca/decguide.html, you can access worksheets to figure out what matters most to you.

More prostate surgery. Prostate cancer often presents men with difficult decisions, because in many cases, it's not clear whether it's better to have surgery or radiation—or just to opt for "watchful waiting." The uncertainty leaves room for doctors to settle on very different approaches. In a scattering of areas in the West, particularly Los Angeles and San Jose in California and the whole of Utah, men are nearly twice as likely to have surgery as those in Connecticut, according to a 2005 study by UCLA researchers.

The reason isn't known, says researcher Tracey L. Krupski, MD, MPH, an assistant professor of surgery at Duke University Medical Center. What is certain: Surgery can cause incontinence and erectile dysfunction—yet it may lengthen life in some cases—so it's a decision that should be made by the patient and physician, not by the luck of the ZIP code.

HOT SPOT: CASPER, WYOMING
Too many back surgeries

Numerous studies have shown that back pain often goes away if you give it enough time, so in much of the country doctors recommend that patients wait it out. But in Casper, surgeons operate. According to 2005 Medicare data, Casper had the highest rate of back surgery in the country—11 per 1,000 Medicare enrollees, more than two and a half times the national average and nearly five times the rate in Vermont and New Jersey.

Researchers aren't sure why people in this city of 50,000 rush to go under the knife, but it may be a classic case of what's known as a "surgical signature": When the best treatment is unclear, local doctors build a consensus. (See "Why Where Matters" on page 37.)

Other hot spots for spine surgery include Boise, Idaho; Great Falls, Montana; and Mason City, Iowa.

Better end-of-life care. The states of Utah and Oregon are seen by many experts as models for restrained but responsible care for terminally ill patients. In a 2006 Dartmouth study that analyzed the records of 4.7 million Medicare patients, the researchers found that people in Utah had an average of just 17 doctor visits in the last 6 months of life, compared with 41.5 visits in New Jersey. Hospital stays were shorter, too: Patients in Utah, Oregon, and Idaho spent an average of 7 to 8 days in the hospital in their final 6 months, roughly half as many as patients in Hawaii, New York, New Jersey, and DC.

Yet less care equaled better care. The Dartmouth researchers found that elderly patients in the West actually lived slightly longer—perhaps because every day in the hospital and each procedure bring risks of infection and other complications.

THE SOUTH

The states: Alabama, Arkansas, Delaware, District of Columbia, Florida, Georgia, Kentucky, Louisiana, Maryland, Mississippi, North Carolina, Oklahoma, South Carolina, Tennessee, Texas, Virginia, and West Virginia

Higher hysterectomy rates. Southern women are more apt than women elsewhere to have their uteruses removed for problems such as fibroids—6.2 per 1,000 women in 2004, compared with 3.7 per 1,000 in the Northeast, according to the most recent data from the CDC. (Rates for the West and Midwest fell in between.) What's more, Southern women lose the organ at age 44, on average, compared with age 49 for women who have the surgery in the Northeast.

"When a woman hears she needs a hysterectomy, she must get more information, wherever she lives," says Michael Broder, MD, an assistant clinical professor of obstetrics and gynecology at UCLA. "It's such a commonly overdone operation."

In a 2000 study, Dr. Broder and colleagues found that 70 percent of hysterectomies at nine medical practices in Southern California were recommended inappropriately: Either the patients weren't adequately evaluated or they weren't offered less invasive options, which include drug therapy and surgery to remove fibroids while sparing the uterus.

Crowded emergency rooms. Because a relatively high number of Southerners lack health insurance, preventive care is hard for many to afford, and that can allow treatable conditions to become emergencies, says Frederick Blum, MD, an emergency physician in Morgantown, West Virginia, and a past president of the American College of Emergency Physicians. The resulting ER overload affects everyone in the state, with victims of car crashes jockeying for medical attention with patients in diabetic shock. In West Virginia, for example, there were 629 emergency room visits per 1,000 residents in 2006, compared with an average of 396 per 1,000 residents across the nation.

Women still take hormones. Use of estrogen supplements—either short-term to treat hot flashes or long-term to protect the bones—has declined dramatically since government studies showed that they can increase the risk of developing breast cancer and heart disease. But the drop-off has been uneven, according to a study released in 2008 by researchers at Express Scripts, a pharmacy benefits manager providing

CHECK YOUR HOSPITAL

Not sure how your local hospital rates? Fortunately, researching the quality of local health care just got easier: The government's revamped Hospital Compare portal now allows you to view patient satisfaction ratings for thousands of hospitals nationwide, and you can find out an institution's safety and success record for a variety of surgeries. You can also check out prices and Medicare reimbursement rates for common procedures, making it easier than ever to evaluate costs at multiple facilities before undergoing an elective operation.

To get started, log on to hospitalcompare.hhs.gov.

services to more than 50 million members.

In Louisiana, the number of women filling estrogen prescriptions shrank about 40 percent from 2000 to 2006—but tumbled a full 74 percent over the same time span in New York. The findings underscore the fact that doctors don't necessarily react to news (or to drug risks) in the same way, so a patient needs to ask questions and be her own advocate.

THE MIDWEST

The states: Illinois, Indiana, Iowa, Kansas, Michigan, Minnesota, Missouri, Nebraska, North Dakota, Ohio, South Dakota, and Wisconsin

Knee surgery rates double. People in the Midwest are prone to knee replacements, according to 2005 Medicare data. The rate in Nebraska was 50 percent higher than the national average—more than double the rate in much of the Northeast. The phenomenon may be partly explained by the greater number of overweight people, who tend to have more knee problems.

But Ronald P. Grelsamer, MD, an orthopedic surgeon and author of several books on knee surgery, suggests that because of the distances Midwestern patients must sometimes travel, physicians may be quicker to offer end-stage treatment when a less invasive one—such as occasional injections—might do the trick.

"With knee replacement, it's a matter of how long a person wants to tough it out before accepting the risks of surgery," he says. That's a decision for the patient, he adds—not the doctor.

Less help for obesity. Midwestern states, along with the South, have the highest rates of morbid obesity in the country. More than 4 percent of women in their fifties weigh so much that they're at greatly increased risk of heart disease and other deadly ills. For them, weight-loss surgery can be lifesaving, says Benjamin Poulose, MD, MPH. But in a 2005 study at Vanderbilt University, he and his colleagues found that those regions had the lowest rates of the surgery: Midwestern or Southern candidates for the surgery were just 25 to 50 percent as likely to get it as those living in the Northeast.

HOT SPOT: ELYRIA, OHIO
Sky-high angioplasty rates

For years, the city of Elyria has had the nation's highest rate of angioplasty, which is a heart treatment that involves threading a balloon catheter through a blocked artery. Local statistics have stood out since at least 1996, according to Dartmouth researchers; by 2003, the city had 42 procedures per 1,000 Medicare enrollees, compared with just 11.3 per 1,000 in the rest of the nation.

A cardiologist's decision to perform angioplasty instead of treating with drugs (or suggesting bypass surgery) is a judgment call in most cases, and the Dartmouth experts say whenever there's that kind of uncertainty, a physician practice or hospital can become wedded to a single approach to the problem.

THE NORTHEAST

The states: Connecticut, Maine, Massachusetts, New Hampshire, New Jersey, New York, Pennsylvania, Rhode Island, and Vermont

Women get better care. Northeastern women get more frequent Pap tests and mammograms than women who live elsewhere in the country. States in the Northeast tend to have patient-friendly policies—ones that boost the number of women with health insurance, for example, or make it easier for workers to take time off to help a family member with medical problems. The result: The region (especially New England) is a good place for women to live, according to a report by the National Women's Law Center and Oregon Health and Science University, which rated states on nearly 100 factors.

"They've put resources into improving the health of their populace, and that pays off," says Michelle Berlin, MD, MPH, an author of the report.

Patients spend an extra 16 percent. Northeasterners tend to see more doctors (including pricey specialists) and get more tests than people in other parts of the country, and they feel it in the pocketbook. Annual costs per person totaled $6,171 in the Northeast in 2004, compared with a national average of $5,283, according to a report by the Centers for Medicare and Medicaid Services.

But that extra care isn't necessarily a good thing, says Elliott Fisher, MD, MPH, a researcher at the Dartmouth Institute. In a 2006 study, patients who saw appreciably more doctors were actually slightly more likely to die, probably because of complications that can accompany procedures and similar factors. Surprisingly, says Dr. Fisher, "the evidence suggests that higher spending is actually associated with lower quality."

fast fact --

15: The millions of incidents of medical harm that occur in US hospitals each year

----

HOT SPOT: NEWARK, NEW JERSEY
Over-hospitalization

Most people hope to spend their final days at home or in a hospice, but in Newark, nearly 50 percent of elderly patients die in a hospital, the most expensive and impersonal way to go. It's the highest rate in the country, according to a review of Medicare data from the mid-1990s. (In Bend, Oregon, where rates are among the lowest in the United States, fewer than 20 percent of Medicare deaths were in a hospital.)

One possible reason: Newark has a lot of hospital beds for a town of its size, and studies show that can affect doctors' behavior. "The more hospital beds there are, the more likely a person will be hospitalized rather than treated at home," says Elliott Fisher, MD, MPH, a researcher at the Dartmouth Institute. "It's easier for the physician, but it's not always best for the patient."

Breast cancer surgery may be less invasive. Although numerous studies have shown virtually equal survival rates for women who get breast-conserving lumpectomy versus those who have a mastectomy, treatment varies significantly from state to state. In a 2006 study at the University of Louisville, 71 percent of breast cancer patients in the Northeast had a lumpectomy, compared with just 63 percent of women in the Southeast.

How a doctor presents the options can tilt a woman's decision, says E. Dale Collins, MD, medical director of the Comprehensive Breast Program at Dartmouth-Hitchcock Medical Center in Lebanon, New Hampshire. So can other factors, including how easy or difficult it is to get follow-up care. Most lumpectomy patients need multiple radiation treatments, she points out, and in some other areas of the country, you might have to drive 2 hours a day to get it. "That might change your treatment choice," she says.

WHY WHERE MATTERS

Of course, location isn't the only factor that impacts the quality of health care, but it certainly is one of the most important. Here, researchers explain the reasons why location determines care.

If you build it, they will come. You'd think that the number of people who need hospital care in an area would determine the number of hospital beds, but it seems to be the other way around. Boston has about 60 percent more hospital beds per person than New Haven, Connecticut, and researchers have found that Bostonians are about 60 percent more likely to be hospitalized, though they're no sicker.

"As we build capacity in the health care system—more hospital beds, more MRI machines—we use it," says Dr. Weinstein. Disturbingly, studies show the quality of health care is somewhat worse in higher-spending regions, maybe because, in terms of infections, a hospital is not a healthy place to be.

FINDING THE WORDS

Telling your doctor you want to see someone else for a second opinion can be awkward, particularly if you've known your doctor for years. But a good physician won't be insulted, and many will recommend it to you themselves. If they don't, here's what you can say (or not say) to your doctor, says Kate Clay, RN, program director at the Center for Shared Decision Making, Dartmouth-Hitchcock Medical Center in Lebanon, New Hampshire.

SAY: "This is a difficult decision for me, and I'd like to learn about other treatments than the one we've discussed. Can you recommend someone I can talk to?"

DON'T SAY: Any version of "I don't trust your judgment. I don't like you. I'm not sure whether you're a good doctor." Comments like these would put anyone on the defensive.

Doctors agree to agree. For certain conditions, there's very little variation in treatment: If you have a hip fracture, you need surgery, wherever you live. But for many ailments, the evidence for a particular treatment is not so clear, which leaves room for lots of variation. Often, though, doctors who work together eventually build a consensus. "Surgical signatures," as the phenomenon is called, may develop as young doctors mimic the practices of their mentors or as they discuss cases over cafeteria lunches. So while physicians in one region may tend toward watchful waiting in the treatment of prostate cancer, for example, those in another area may feel that more aggressive treatment is warranted.

Plain old profit. The sorry fact is that sometimes doctors recommend a treatment because it's more profitable. Physicians who have a financial interest in an imaging center, for example, may be tempted to suggest an MRI even when it's not absolutely necessary.

Sometimes, they recommend much more than an exam: A few years ago, Tenet Healthcare Corporation agreed to pay more than $50 million (without admitting fault) to settle government charges that doctors at the Redding Medical Center in Redding, California, performed unnecessary heart procedures and surgeries on hundreds of patients.

fast fact ---

Hospitals that participate in clinical trials provide better care to cardiac patients and have lower death rates due to heart attacks than nonparticipating hospitals. A study found that the mortality rate for nonparticipating hospitals was 5.9 percent, while the rate for hospitals with low participation was 4.4 percent. The death rate for hospitals actively involved in trials was 3.5 percent.

The results show that patients treated at participating hospitals received better care and more positive outcomes. The researchers say successful clinical trials rely on physicians with leadership skills, common goals, open and credible feedback, and strong administrative support. These are also the characteristics that make for a high-quality hospital.

HEALTH HEROES

When tragedy strikes, she helps patients pick up the pieces

In 1999, Linda Kenney, from Mansfield, Massachusetts, went in for routine ankle surgery; an anesthesia mishap caused her heart to stop, and she nearly died. Worse, the lawsuit-fearing hospital wouldn't tell her what went wrong. She started Medically Induced Trauma Support Services (MITSS) to get patients and hospitals talking—to mend fences without the threat of litigation. The organization provides counseling and help finding answers. "It's a great comfort to hear your doctor is sorry," she says.

For more information, visit the MITSS Web site www.mitss.org.

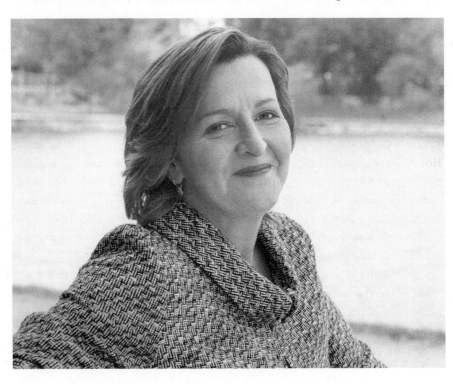

GET PAIN RELIEF—STAT

Research proves that some natural remedies can be just as good at beating pain than medications

You're in pain, and ibuprofen just won't cut it. NSAIDs don't agree with your stomach, and you're wary of stronger meds. But you just don't have time for this pain; you're desperate to feel better—fast.

Fortunately, you have alternatives—natural ones. From herbs that attack inflammation to techniques that leverage the brain's remarkable healing powers to a simple trick to ward off "needle stick" pains, nature offers many treatments for conditions such as arthritis, fibromyalgia, and even muscle strains.

Here are eight natural remedies that may enhance or replace conventional antidotes, and they'll leave you happier, healthier, and pain free.

CAPSAICIN

What it's for: Arthritis, shingles, or neuropathy

What the science says: An active component of chile pepper, capsaicin temporarily desensitizes pain-prone skin nerve receptors called C-fibers; soreness is diminished for 3 to 5 weeks while they regain sensation. Nearly 40 percent of people with arthritis reduced their pain by half after using a topical capsaicin cream for a month, and 60 percent of people with neuropathy achieved the same after 2 months, according to a University of Oxford study. Patients at the New England Center for Headache in Stamford, Connecticut, decreased their migraine and cluster headache intensity after applying capsaicin cream inside their nostrils.

How to try it: Capsaicin ointments and creams are sold in pharmacies and health food stores. For arthritis or neuropathy, try 0.025 percent or 0.075 percent capsaicin cream one to four times daily; best results can take up to 2 weeks, says Philip Gregory, PharmD, a professor at Creighton University and editor of the Natural Medicines Comprehensive Database. But research on capsaicin and headaches remains limited, and don't expect stronger versions anytime soon. "Current formulations are better suited for more acute problems, like a sore muscle or an arthritis flare-up, than everyday pain and stiffness," Gregory says.

INFLATHERA OR ZYFLAMEND

What it's for: Arthritis

What the science says: Both supplement brands contain ginger, turmeric, and holy basil, all of which have anti-inflammatory properties. Turmeric (a curry ingredient) may be the best: A component, curcumin, eases inflammatory conditions such as rheumatoid arthritis (RA) and psoriasis, according to the Methodist Research Institute in Indianapolis. Researchers are now testing Zyflamend in RA patients, but some experts are already sold: "Each herb has its own scientific database of evidence," says James Dillard, MD, author of *The Chronic Pain Solution*.

How to try it: ProThera, InflaThera's maker, will only sell to health care professionals, so your doctor has to order it for you; that said, it's reportedly stronger (and slightly cheaper) than Zyflamend. InflaThera's suggested dosage is twice daily with food. For the more readily accessible Zyflamend, take one capsule two or three times daily, but avoid it near bedtime—each pill contains 10 milligrams of caffeine (another version, Zyflamend PM, is reportedly less stimulating). You can buy Zyflamend at swansonvitamins.com or prohealth.com/zyflamend.htm.

Or save money and try curcumin to start: Taking 500 milligrams four times daily, along with fish oil and a diet low in animal fat, can ease arthritis, says Jane Guiltinan, ND, immediate past president of the American Association of Naturopathic Physicians.

ARNICA

What it's for: Acute injury or postsurgery swelling

What the science says: This herb comes from a European flower; although its healing mechanism is still unknown, it does have natural anti-inflammatory properties. Taking oral homeopathic arnica after a tonsillectomy decreases pain, say British researchers, and German doctors found that it reduces surgery-related knee swelling.

How to try it: Use homeopathic arnica as an adjunct to ice, herbs, or conventional pain meds, suggests Guiltinan. Rub arnica ointment on bruises or strained muscles, or take it in the form of three lactose pellets under the tongue up to six times per day. Boiron (boironusa.com) is among the most reputable arnica manufacturers.

AQUAMIN

What it's for: Osteoarthritis

What the science says: This red seaweed supplement is rich in calcium and magnesium. A preliminary clinical study showed that the ingredients may reduce joint inflammation or even help build bone, says David O'Leary of Marigot, Aquamin's Irish manufacturer. In a study of 70 volunteers published in *Nutrition Journal*, Aquamin users reduced arthritis pain by 20 percent in a month and had less stiffness than people taking a placebo.

How to try it: Marigot recommends 2,400 milligrams a day (two capsules) of Aquamin in tablet form, sold domestically in products such as Aquamin Sea Minerals and Cal-Sea-Um. A 60-pill jar of Swanson Vegetarian Aquamin Sea Minerals costs about $6 at swansonvitamins.com.

SAM-E (S-ADENOSYLMETHIONINE)

What it's for: Osteoarthritis

What the science says: SAM-e is made from a naturally occurring amino acid and sold as capsules. Doctors aren't entirely sure why it tamps down pain, but it reduces inflammation and may increase the feel-good brain chemicals serotonin and dopamine. Studies by the University of Maryland School of Nursing and the University of California, Irvine, showed that SAM-e was as effective as some NSAIDs in easing osteoarthritis aches; the California researchers found that SAM-e quashed pain by 50 percent after 2 months, though it took a few weeks to kick in. SAM-e produced no cardiovascular risks and fewer stomach problems than the conventional meds.

How to try it: Costco and CVS both carry it; a month's supply costs $30 to $60. Guiltinan prescribes 400 to 1,600 milligrams daily, often with turmeric or fish oil. SAM-e can interact with other meds, especially MAO-inhibitor antidepressants, so it's vital to talk with your doctor before taking it (and avoid SAM-e entirely if you have bipolar disorder).

Also, inspect the packaging before buying, advises Gregory: Make sure the product carries a USP or GMP quality seal, contains a stabilizing salt, has a far-off expiration date, and comes in foil blister packs because SAM-e can degrade rapidly in direct light.

FISH OIL

What it's for: Joint pain from arthritis or autoimmune disorders

What the science says: Digested fish oil breaks down into hormone-like chemicals called prostaglandins, which reduce inflammation. In one study, about 40 percent of rheumatoid arthritis patients who took cod-liver oil every day were able to cut their NSAID use by more than one-third, Scottish scientists reported.

People with neck and back pain have fared even better: After about 10 weeks, nearly two-thirds were able to stop taking NSAIDs altogether in a University of Pittsburgh study.

How to try it: Taking 1,000 milligrams is proven to help your heart, but you should up the dose for pain. For osteoarthritis, try 2,000 to 4,000 milligrams daily; for rheumatoid arthritis and autoimmune diseases associated with joint pain (such as lupus), consider a much higher dose of upwards

JUST A FISH STORY?

Still think most omega-3 product claims sound, well, downright fishy? The truth is they're probably a good catch after all. A ConsumerLab.com analysis of 49 popular fish-oil products found that all of them contained their claimed amounts of omega-3 fatty acids DHA and EPA (which can lower blood pressure, reduce inflammation, and even grow new brain cells). None had unsafe mercury levels. One supplement (Kirkland brand) released its fish oil too quickly, the study found—making for some aromatic burps, at most—but few other problems were reported.

of 8,000 milligrams daily, but ask your doctor about such a large amount first, says Tanya Edwards, MD, medical director at the Cleveland Clinic's Center for Integrative Medicine. (The same rule applies if you take blood pressure or heart medications, because omega-3s can thin the blood.)

Read the nutrition label carefully: The dosage refers to the amount of omega-3s that's in a capsule, not other ingredients. Nordic Naturals (nordicnaturals.com) and Carlson (carlsonlabs.com) are both reputable brands; for something stronger, GNC's Triple-Strength Fish Oil (gnc.com) has 900 milligrams of omega-3s per capsule.

METHYLSULFONYLMETHANE (MSM)

What it's for: Osteoarthritis

What the science says: MSM is derived from sulfur and may prevent joint and cartilage degeneration, say University of California, San Diego, scientists. People with osteoarthritis of the knee who took MSM had 25 percent less pain and 30 percent better physical function at the end of a 3-month trial at Southwest College of Naturopathic Medicine and Health Sciences. Indian researchers also found that MSM worked better when combined with glucosamine.

How to try it: Start with 1.5 to 3 grams once daily and increase to 3 grams twice daily for more severe pain, suggests Leslie Axelrod, ND, a professor of clinical sciences at Southwest College. Patients in the Indian trial improved on dosages as low as 500 milligrams three times daily. Vendors of OptiMSM, the brand tested in Axelrod's trial, can be found at optimsm.com.

COUNTING OUT LOUD

What it's for: Brief "needle stick" pain

What the science says: Patients who counted backward from 100 out loud during an injection experienced and recalled less pain, according to a Japanese study. None of the 46 patients who counted complained

MIX-AND-MATCH PAIN RELIEF

We asked two MDs and two NDs to name their favorite natural pain-reliever and supplement combos, for even more ache-easing efficacy.

FOR ARTHRITIS, TRY: Capsaicin ointment (one to three times daily) + Boswellia, a tree herb (60 percent concentration, 250 milligrams three times daily) + curcumin (400 to 600 milligrams three times daily)

OR: Capsaicin (two or three times daily) + acupuncture (one or two times weekly) + fish oil (1,000 to 8,000 milligrams daily) + magnesium (500 to 1,000 milligrams daily) + vitamin D (1,000 to 5,000 IU daily)

OR: Zyflamend (two or three capsules daily) + fish oil (1,000 to 3,000 milligrams daily) + acupuncture (one or two times weekly) for 1 month

FOR ARTHRITIS OR FIBROMYALGIA, TRY: Fish oil (1,000 to 8,000 milligrams daily) + vitamin D (1,000 to 5,000 IU daily) + magnesium (500 to 1,000 milligrams daily)

OR: SAM-e (400 to 1,500 milligrams daily) + curcumin (500 milligrams three or four times daily) + fish oil (1,000 to 3,000 milligrams daily)

OR: Curcumin (1,000 to 2,000 milligrams daily) + fish oil (1,000 to 8,000 milligrams daily)

Always ask your doctor before starting any new supplements. Efficacy and response time for all therapies can vary by individual.

afterward, and only one of them could remember pain from the injection at all (among the 46 who didn't count, 19 said the injection hurt and 10 recalled what it felt like).

Recitation might work by distracting the brain from processing the sensation, says study author Tomoko Higashi, MD, of Yokohama City University Medical Center in Kanagawa, Japan. The trick is probably only useful for short or acute periods, she says, adding: "The degree of pain reduction really depends on how well patients concentrate on counting."

BOOST YOUR HEALTH THE EASY WAY

Studies show that small tweaks in lifestyle can reap healthy rewards

Perfectionism may seem like a desirable trait, but to boost your health, aim for "just enough." "Trying to do everything right promotes an all-or-nothing attitude," says Martin Binks, PhD, a psychologist at the Duke Diet and Fitness Center in Durham, North Carolina. So if you can't do something perfectly (such as working out an hour a day), you don't do anything at all (such as watching TV instead). A better mind-set: Believe that every little bit counts. "It's small changes that are most effective," Binks says. So forget perfect!

Here, the "good enough" guidelines for nine common get-healthy recommendations that will ensure you're on your way to a longer, disease-free life.

FRUITS AND VEGETABLES

Gold standard: Up to 9 servings of fruits and vegetables a day

Good enough: Five a day

That's all it took for men and women to lower their stroke risk by 31 percent, according to a Harvard University study. "Five servings provide significant antioxidants and fiber to reduce heart disease and cancer risk and keep your weight in check," says Rosa Mo, RD, a nutrition professor at the University of New Haven. (One serving is equivalent to one medium piece of fresh fruit, ½ cup of cut fruit, 1 cup of raw leafy greens, or ½ cup of other cooked vegetables, such as broccoli.)

Boost the benefit: Keep 'em cool and eat a rainbow of colors. Refrigerating berries, citrus, and fruit with edible skin (think apples), as well as veggies, preserves antioxidants. And aiming to eat from at least three different color groups (such as green, orange/yellow, red, white, and blue/purple) a day will ensure you get a wide variety of nutrients.

EXERCISE

Gold standard: 30 minutes of cardio 5 or more days a week

Good enough: 17 minutes a day

A study from Brigham and Women's Hospital in Boston found that women who exercised just 2 hours a week (or 17 minutes daily) reduced their risk of heart disease and stroke by 27 percent.

"You don't even have to do it all at once. No fewer than 10 studies since 1995 show that breaking up physical activity into small segments of about 10 minutes is just as effective," says Barry Franklin, PhD, director of cardiac rehabilitation and exercise laboratories at Beaumont Hospital in Royal Oak, Michigan, and spokesperson for the American Heart Association's national "Start!" program.

Boost the benefit: Pick up your pace for 30 to 60 seconds several times during your workout. A study from McMaster University in Canada found that people who did a total of 2 to 3 minutes of high-intensity exercise in the form of 30-second all-out sprints improved their cardiovascular fitness and muscle endurance as much as those who did 40 to 60 minutes of moderate-intensity exercise.

SUNSCREEN

Gold standard: Apply SPF 30 or higher several times a day

Good enough: Put it on first thing in the morning

"Most women don't put on any sunscreen, so this is a huge improvement that can decrease your risk of both skin cancer and skin damage," says Doris J. Day, MD, a clinical assistant professor of dermatology at New York University Medical Center. SPF 15 blocks 93 percent of rays, compared with 97 percent for SPF 30 (which also lasts longer). Unless you're spending the day poolside, put a moisturizer with at least SPF 30 on your face, neck, chest, hands, and any other exposed areas in the morning.

Boost the benefit: Reapply sunscreen before you go out for lunch, when the sun's rays are strongest. Dr. Day recommends Colorescience's Sunforgettable ($50; colorescience.com for store locations), a colorless powder with an SPF 30 that easily goes over your makeup in just 5 seconds. (You can use it on other body parts, too.)

STAYING HYDRATED

Gold standard: Eight 8-ounce glasses of water daily

Good enough: Drink with meals and when you're thirsty

Sipping water isn't the only way to stay hydrated. Other beverages (including caffeinated options such as coffee and tea) and foods that contain water (such as soup and fresh fruits and vegetables) contribute, too. In fact, food makes up about 20 percent of your water intake daily. A National Academy of Sciences panel determined that healthy women get adequate amounts of fluids (an average of 11 glasses a day) from normal drinking habits such as having beverages with meals, through the foods they eat, and by letting their thirst guide them. (The exception: Active women and those living in hot climates may have to make a concerted effort to stay hydrated.)

Boost the benefit: Gulp before you eat. A study from Virginia Polytechnic Institute and State University found that people who drank 1½ cups of water prior to eating a meal reported feeling fuller and, as a result, consumed about 60 fewer calories than those who didn't drink beforehand.

SLEEP

Gold standard: 8 hours a night
Good enough: 7 hours

You may feel less than peppy the next day, but you won't be putting your health at risk, says Susan Zafarlotfi, PhD, director of the Institute of Sleep/Wake Disorders Clinic at Hackensack University Medical Center in New Jersey.

But less than that and you might: Research is turning up links between inadequate sleep and heart disease, hypertension, diabetes, and obesity. A study from Case Western Reserve University of about 68,000 middle-age women found that those who slept 5 or fewer hours were 32 percent more likely to experience major weight gain, and 15 percent more likely to become obese, than those who slept an average of 7 hours.

KITCHEN CURE

Want a good night's sleep and to slow down aging? Sniff some lavender. The scent will bring you a restful sleep, and studies show it can also reduce levels of cortisol, the hormone that increases blood pressure and suppresses the immune system. What's more, it appears to help rid the body of free radicals, those pesky molecules believed to speed aging and disease. (Surprised that this is a Kitchen Cure? Yes, you can eat lavender; the delicate flowers are edible.)

"Sleeping less than 6 hours even just a few nights has been tied to poorer decision making and reduced alertness," says Zafarlotfi. Make it a habit and your risks of diabetes and depression increase, too.

Boost the benefit: Slip on socks. Warm feet widen blood vessels, which better enables your body to transfer heat so you sleep more soundly. And turn your alarm clock away from you. Light signals your brain to wake up, and the "blue light" from your digital clock and cell phone are the worst offenders.

PORTION SIZES

Gold standard: Measure everything you eat

Good enough: Size up grains and fats only

"Few people become obese eating lots of fruits and vegetables," says Mo. On the other hand, grains (such as bread, rice, pasta, and cereal) and fats (such as nuts, butter, oil, avocado, and salad dressing) tend to be more calorie dense, advises Mo. Doubling up on these types of foods can quickly add to your total calorie intake, while extra-large portions of fruits and veggies do less damage, and their high fiber content makes it hard to overeat them.

Boost the benefit: To naturally cut back on calories, start lunch or dinner with one or two baseball-size servings of high-fiber water-filled vegetables (such as steamed cauliflower, broccoli, or spinach). "You'll be less likely to overeat the more calorie-rich foods in your meal because you'll already feel full," Mo says.

STRENGTH TRAINING

Gold standard: Two or three times a week

Good enough: Once a week

Research shows that people who lifted weights weekly for 2 months gained nearly as much lean muscle (about 3 pounds) as those who worked out three times a week. "It took them several weeks longer, but the results were similar," says Wayne Westcott, PhD, fitness research director at the South Shore YMCA in Quincy, Massachusetts, and coauthor of *Get Stronger, Feel Younger.*

Boost the benefit: Slow down! Taking your time with each lift builds muscle faster. Allow 3 to 4 seconds to lift or contract a muscle (such as raising a dumbbell during a biceps curl), and 3 to 4 seconds to release or lower the weight.

WASHING YOUR HANDS

Gold standard: Lather for at least 15 to 20 seconds before rinsing
Good enough: Wash for 10 seconds, then rinse

A study from the University of North Carolina at Chapel Hill shows that's enough to knock off more than 90 percent of infection-causing microbes. "The length of time is less important than simply doing it regularly—especially after you use the bathroom, touch someone who's ill, or handle raw meat or unwashed vegetables," says Paul Lyons, MD, an associate professor of family and community medicine at Temple University School of Medicine. "You don't have to be stringent about technique either; just create a lather and rinse thoroughly."

Boost the benefit: Skip the antibacterial soap. Regular soap and water is not only just as effective, but it may actually be better for your health, too. "Some research suggests that overuse of antibacterial soaps may contribute to the development of super-resistant strains of bacteria," explains Diana Noah, PhD, an infectious disease expert with the Southern Research Institute, a nonprofit health research organization in Birmingham, Alabama.

A HEALTHY WEIGHT

Gold standard: BMI between 19 and 25
Good enough: Aim to lose 5 to 7 percent of your current body weight
That's equivalent to 8 to 11 pounds if you're 5-foot-4 and 165 pounds.

Although, according to a BMI scale, you're still in the overweight category, a National Institutes of Health study found that weight loss in this range can reduce your risk of diabetes by 58 percent.

"Numerous other studies show that it's also enough to lower blood pressure and cholesterol as well as risk of heart disease," says David Arterburn, MD, MPH, an obesity researcher at the Group Health Center for Health Studies at the University of Washington.

Boost the benefit: Exercise and eat MUFAs. More commonly known as monounsaturated fatty acids, these healthy dietary fats, found in olive oil, nuts, and avocado, can help you shed some of the most dangerous body fat—the disease-promoting kind around your middle. And dieters who also exercise lose up to 57 percent more belly fat than those who aren't active.

BUST SOME MYTHS

Science disproves some of the most popular (and persistent) health rumors

Does reading in low light really hurt your eyes? How about sitting too close to the TV? (No, and no.) Why are you better off drinking exactly eight glasses of water per day? (You're not.) Does your body burn more calories digesting ice cold beverages and food? (Yes, hurray!) Thanks to quack culture, the Internet, and well-intentioned but poorly informed relatives, it's become harder than ever to separate fact from fiction. Whatever its origin, misleading health information can cause unnecessary anxiety and distract you from wellness habits that truly deserve your energy and attention. Here's a dissection of several watercooler myths that will give you all the authority you need to refute your brother's latest forwarded e-mails.

NONSTICK PANS CAUSE CANCER

The verdict: Jury's out

The chemical behind this scare is perfluorooctanoic acid, or PFOA, which is a substance used to make nonstick coating. In animals, high levels of PFOA have been linked to cancer, low birth weight, and other health problems. This chemical is also found in stain-resistant carpets, pizza boxes, and microwave popcorn bags.

Human studies are limited, but at least 90 percent of Americans have small amounts of PFOA in their bloodstreams, and it can linger for years, says Kristina Thayer, PhD, deputy director of the Office of Risk Assessment Research at the National Institute of Environmental Health Sciences (NIEHS), who has reviewed the research on this topic. DuPont, the company that manufactures the Teflon brand, recommends cooking at a maximum temperature of 500°F (medium-high); at temperatures higher than 660°F, the coating can start to break down and possibly release PFOA and other toxic gases.

The bottom line: Add water or oil to a nonstick pan when you turn on the flame to absorb the heat and never raise temps above medium-high. Because PFOA can escape when the nonstick surface degrades, toss the pan if you see scratches or particles flaking into food.

ALUMINUM CAUSES ALZHEIMER'S DISEASE

The verdict: Not likely

This concern took root in the 1960s, when studies on animals showed that exposing them to this metal produced nerve damage similar to that found in Alzheimer's patients. In humans, some studies found increased aluminum levels in the brains of Alzheimer's patients, but the metal itself doesn't cause the disease, says John Trojanowski, MD, PhD, director of the Institute on Aging and the Alzheimer's Disease Core Center at the University of Pennsylvania. He has authored more than 350 studies on Alzheimer's.

Absorbing more than 1,000 milligrams of aluminum per day may be toxic to the brain, but the average person who cooks with aluminum pans, wraps leftovers in foil, and drinks from cans ingests 9 milligrams at most, says Maria Carrillo, PhD, director of medical and scientific relations at the Alzheimer's Association.

The bottom line: Although aluminum has science's seal of approval, cast- or rolled-iron pans are an even healthier option. They safely impart iron, which is an essential nutrient, into food.

HEATING PLASTIC IN THE MICROWAVE CAUSES CANCER

The verdict: Jury's out

Experts say it's better to use glass or paper towels in the microwave. Some studies in rodents have tied plasticizers (chemicals that make plastic soft and pliable) to cancer and developmental disorders.

Still, this doesn't mean you should ban plastic containers from your home, says Ted Widlanski, PhD, of Indiana University, who's led several studies examining the possible cancer link. Certain plasticizers from containers and plastic wrap can migrate into food at room temperature, but heat speeds the process significantly, says Paul Blanc, MD, chief of the Division of Occupational and Environmental Medicine at the University of California, San Francisco.

The bottom line: Nuke only containers labeled "microwave safe"; others can break down or melt when heated, Dr. Blanc says. Even better, choose Rubbermaid and Tupperware bowls. These were deemed 100 percent safe in a *Consumer Reports* study. No trace of chemicals was found in food after heating.

THE 5-SECOND RULE IS SAFE

The Verdict: Fiction

It's probably not even safe to follow a 1-second rule: The transfer of bacteria from a contaminated surface to food is almost instantaneous— or, at the very least, quicker than your reflexes. In a recent study, Clemson University food scientist Paul Dawson, PhD, and students contaminated several surfaces (ceramic tile, wood flooring, and carpet) with salmonella. They then dropped pieces of bologna and slices of bread on the surfaces for as little as 5 seconds and as long as 60 seconds. After just 5 seconds, both food types had already picked up as many as 1,800 bacteria (more bad bugs adhered to the moisture-rich bologna than to the bread). After a full minute, it was up to 10 times that amount.

The bottom line: There are 76 million cases of foodborne illness annually in the United States, according to the Centers for Disease Control and Prevention, so unless you're the only family on the block that sterilizes their floors on an hourly basis, you should refrain from eating dropped food.

"Let's not forget what comes into contact with floors—people bring animal feces on their shoes into their homes," Dawson says. And don't assume that countertops are clean. As last year's tomato-related illnesses nationwide showed, "raw fruits and vegetables are as frequently the perpetrators of salmonella transfer as poultry," Dawson says.

CRACKING YOUR KNUCKLES CAUSES ARTHRITIS

The Verdict: Fiction

If you're suffering from osteoarthritis in your hands, it certainly has nothing to do with this nervous tic. One study at the former Mount Carmel Mercy Hospital in Detroit compared 74 people (age 45 and older) who had been chronic knuckle crackers for decades with 226 who always left their hands alone; researchers found no difference in the incidence of osteoarthritis between the two groups.

But there are reasons to stop this annoying habit: The same study found knuckle crackers to be far more likely to have weaker grip strength and greater hand swelling, both of which can limit dexterity. As for osteo-arthritis, that's more likely due to genetics and increasing age.

The bottom line: Try channeling your nervous energy into a less harmful habit that occupies your hands—such as doodling. If a different activity doesn't get you to stop, try putting a large rubber band around your wrist and every time you catch yourself cracking your knuckles, pull it back and let it snap as a reminder that your habit can be harmful. Most important, get to the bottom of what's causing your nervousness in the first place. You may discover that you crack your knuckles more often at work than at home, for example. Address those sources directly.

COLA-TYPE DRINKS DAMAGE YOUR KIDNEYS

The verdict: Fact

Despite their global popularity, there's nothing remotely healthy about cola beverages: Drinking 16 ounces or more daily (whether diet or regular) doubles your risk of chronic kidney disease, according to a National Institutes of Health (NIH) study of more than 900 people. The researchers already knew that consuming any type of soft drink is associated with several risk factors for kidney disease (hypertension, diabetes, and kidney stones), but the spike in the cola category was remarkable. Experts suspect that the ingredient phosphoric acid may be the culprit; it's been repeatedly linked to "urinary changes that promote kidney stones," say the study authors.

Cola has an additional knock against it: Consumption is associated with significantly lower bone density in women, increasing the risk of osteoporosis and bone fractures, says a separate study.

The bottom line: If you're going to indulge in an occasional soda, go

fast fact --
The average American adult guzzles 59 gallons' worth of cola drinks each year. That's one big gulp.
----

for Sprite, 7-Up, ginger ale, and the like. The NIH study found that non-cola drinks didn't have the same impact on the kidneys. But you'll be better off if you skip soda altogether, even the sugar-free varieties: Recent research showed a link between drinking diet soda and weight gain.

PLASTIC WATER BOTTLES LEACH DANGEROUS CHEMICALS

The verdict: Jury's out

Experts aren't sure whether plastic bottles are safe. Although there's no conclusive evidence that chemicals in these disposable bottles transfer into the water, experts say possible health risks are big enough to make you think twice.

One danger is that they might be formulated with a chemical called bisphenol-A (BPA): It behaves like estrogen and can disturb the endocrine system, says Frederick vom Saal, PhD, a leading researcher on BPA at the University of Missouri–Columbia. There's no way to know whether a disposable water bottle contains it, but scientists know one type of bottle

THE SQUEEZE TEST

If you're not sure whether your water bottle is made with a chemical called bisphenol-A (BPA), give it a squeeze. If the bottle doesn't give, it's almost certainly made with this chemical.

Single-use water bottles are generally made from a safer plastic: polyethylene terephthalate (PETE or PET), designated by a number 1 in the recycling sign found on the bottle's bottom. However, those bottles can leach other chemicals, called phthalates, which are also thought to be endocrine disruptors.

The safest option is to get your water from the tap or, if you want to take it with you, put it in a metal sports bottle.

does: the reusable, hard plastic kind, usually found in sporting goods stores for hikers, bikers, and weekend soccer players. Rodents exposed to similar doses of the chemicals as humans receive when they drink from these bottles had higher rates of breast cancer, early onset puberty, reduced sperm counts, and neurological disorders, found a 2006 review of 700 studies by the NIEHS.

The bottom line: Bottled water is convenient, but if the unknowns worry you, switch to tap water (filtered, if you prefer), and replace your sports bottle with a stainless-steel version.

YOUR BODY BURNS MORE CALORIES DIGESTING ICY BEVERAGES AND FOODS

The verdict: Fact

But before you give yourself an ice-cream headache, there's more. "The small difference in calories probably won't make a significant dent in your diet," explains Madelyn Fernstrom, PhD, founding director of the Weight Management Center at the University of Pittsburgh Medical Center. On the bright side, different studies have suggested that five or six ice-cold glasses of water could help you burn about 10 extra calories a day— equaling about 1 pound of nearly effortless weight loss every year.

The bottom line: Although the metabolism-boosting effects are small, it can't hurt to pour no-cal drinks—water, tea, coffee—on the rocks to maximize your body's calorie-burning potential.

EATING GRAPEFRUIT SPEEDS METABOLISM

The verdict: Fiction

Grapefruit won't work miracles for your metabolism, but it can help you lose weight. Half a grapefruit before meals helped individuals lose about 4 pounds in 12 weeks, according to a study published in the *Journal of Medicinal Food*. The reason: Its fiber and water fill you up on fewer calories, so you eat less at your next meal.

The bottom line: Be sure to include this tangy fruit in your diet—not because it burns calories, but because it's flavorful, nutritious, and satisfying.

"DOUBLE-DIPPING" SPREADS GERMS

The verdict: Fact

In a classic episode of *Seinfeld*, a partygoer accused George Costanza of spreading germs by "double-dipping"—swiping a chip into a bowl of dip, taking a bite, and then dipping the same chip again.

Having settled the 5-second rule debate, Clemson University's Dawson decided to do the same with this alleged party faux pas. It turns out that George really was contaminating the other guests: Using Wheat Thins and various dips, Dawson found that a double-dip deposited thousands of saliva bacteria into the dip—and of those, 50 to 100 were later transferred through the dip to a clean cracker, presumably destined for another guest's mouth. Still unknown, however, is how long such bacteria can survive in the dip or whether they can actually infect another dipper upon ingestion.

The bottom line: You'd better be pretty comfy with your party guests. "Eating from a dip after someone has dipped twice is basically the same as kissing that person," Dawson says. Be especially wary of thin dips; the study found that the lower the dip's viscosity, the higher the rate of germ transfer from a double-dip. For example, a chip's second plunge into a cheese dip is less cause for concern than a watery salsa. Thicker dips apparently don't allow errant bacteria to travel as far as thinner varieties do. Finally, think twice about digging into any dip at the end of the night; remnants on the sides or bottom of a bowl are most likely a highly concentrated mash of germs, Dawson says, akin to the last sip in a can of soda.

LOCALLY PRODUCED HONEY EASES HAY FEVER

The verdict: Jury's out

The theory seems sound: Bees in your neighborhood feed on the same pollen that gives you itchy eyes and a runny nose. That pollen gets added to the hive's honey, and ingesting it helps you build a tolerance to those allergens—or so the thinking goes. But does this really work?

"We don't know—there are no studies to support it, only testimonials," says Leonard Bielory, MD, director of the Asthma and Allergy Research Center at the New Jersey Medical School. Of course, the same process could produce negative effects. Bees may visit problem plants, such as poison ivy, and cause a rash in people ingesting the ivy-tainted honey. Yet anecdotal reports claim just the opposite: Some honey lovers insist that the sweetener has helped build an immunity to such reactions.

The bottom line: Keep standard allergy remedies on hand, but feel free to enjoy local honey, too. It's a worthy replacement for other sweeteners and even has natural antibiotic properties.

CELL PHONES INTERFERE WITH HOSPITALS' MEDICAL EQUIPMENT

The verdict: Jury's out

There's a chance that a cell phone call in the wrong spot can cause ventilators, syringe pumps, or even pacemakers to pulse incorrectly, according to a 2007 Dutch study. The researchers tested modern cell phones, including PDAs that use wireless Internet signals. After placing the phones just a couple of inches from devices, researchers found that 43 percent of the phones caused electromagnetic interference with critical care equipment—and a third of those instances could be potentially life-threatening to patients.

But those findings countered a Mayo Clinic study a year prior that found no instances of "clinically important" interference between cell phones and medical machines. In fact, Mayo researchers advised hospitals to revise or drop their cell phone bans.

The bottom line: Play it safe for now: Use a designated cell phone area at the hospital, which most now offer, or use a call as an excuse for a walk-and-talk outside for some fresh air and exercise. If you feel compelled to stay by a relative's side in the ER or recovery room, be sure to carry a good old-fashioned calling card to use at a pay phone.

LIGHT UP YOUR LIFE

The right dose of light
can decrease appetite, boost
concentration, improve mood,
and even resist disease

Many ancient cultures, including the Egyptians and Greeks, worshipped the sun. Turns out, they were on to something. Every morning, light absorbed by your retinas helps set a master clock in your brain that cues other biological timepieces that regulate blood pressure, temperature, and hormone production. Ongoing light stimulation and the lack of it at the end of the day keeps this complex system, known as circadian rhythms, cycling in an orderly fashion.

With a keen understanding of these light-regulated patterns, you can boost energy, alertness, and your defenses against disease. Here are ways to maximize light's benefits that are so new that even your doctor might not know about them.

MORNING

Start the day off light.

Rise and truly shine. First thing upon waking, head for the brightest light available. It's the fastest way to shake off sleepiness. "Without that light boost, your alarm clock might say 7 a.m., but your body will still feel in the dark," says Mariana G. Figueiro, PhD, an assistant professor at the Lighting Research Center at Rensselaer Polytechnic Institute. For extra alertness, don't wear sunglasses during your morning commute.

Have to rise while it's still dark? Try a bedside lamp with a bluish white compact fluorescent bulb, which is similar to morning light and twice as effective at activating the circadian system as warmer incandescent lights. Buy bulbs labeled Daylight or 6500K.

Boost your concentration. Sunlight directly activates the parts of the brain responsible for maintaining alertness. At work, place your desk by a window, if possible, taking care to avoid glare. A work performance study by the California Energy Commission linked working by a window with better concentration and short-term memory recall. In another study of 21,000 students, those in the sunniest classrooms solved math problems 20 percent faster.

Get an energy jolt. The first rays of early morning suppress the production of melatonin (a hormone that makes you feel sleepy) and keep your circadian cycle on track so you feel more alert during the day. To fend off an afternoon energy slump, it's best to take an early morning walk.

"This synchronizes your body clock to your watch and will make you feel more energetic all day, as well as sleep better at night," says Figueiro.

Improve your mood. Light encourages production of serotonin, the mood-regulating neurotransmitter. Insufficient exposure to light, particularly during the short days of the winter months, can lead to mild depression. Consider using a light box made especially for combating seasonal affective disorder (SAD), a condition that affects some people during the darkest days of winter. Look for one featuring blue light-emitting

TIMING IS EVERYTHING

Taking some medications to coincide with the peaks and valleys of your light-regulated body clock can increase their effectiveness. For instance, French researchers found that timed doses of chemotherapy on people with late-stage colorectal cancer outperformed nearly all other treatments. Everyday prescription drugs also work best when synced up with the body rhythms. Always check with your doctor before altering your meds. Here's a breakdown of what works better when.

For Allergies

MEDICATION: Antihistamines

TAKE AT: Bedtime. The active ingredient will be in your bloodstream before symptoms are at their worst in the morning.

For Arthritis

MEDICATION: Long-acting painkillers (Celebrex, Naprelan)

TAKE AT: In the morning for osteoarthritis, with an additional dose at night for rheumatoid arthritis.

For Asthma

MEDICATION: Oral prednisone

TAKE AT: 3 p.m. Research shows it's more effective at controlling nighttime symptoms (which tend to be more severe) than an 8 a.m. dose is. The same study found an 8 p.m. dose was only slightly more effective than a placebo.

For High Blood Pressure

MEDICATION: Hypertension drugs (Covera-HS, Innopran XL)

TAKE AT: Bedtime. This provides highest drug levels in the morning when blood pressure is highest.

For High Cholesterol

MEDICATION: Short-acting statins (Zocor, Lescol)

TAKE AT: Bedtime. Because your body makes cholesterol at night, the drugs reduce cholesterol 30 to 35 percent more effectively than a morning dose does.

diodes (LEDs) with a peak wavelength of 470 nanometers, which are more effective for the circadian system and produce less glare than white-light boxes.

Rein in your appetite. Eons of evolution have programmed our appetite to respond to light in the early morning, when our ancestors needed energy for hard work, and to diminish after dark, when they needed rest. Electric lighting, however, has made it possible for us to stay awake and snack when we used to be sleeping. Even worse, research shows that we also find food less satisfying in the evening, which keeps us noshing.

To put the brakes on nighttime nibbling, eat a substantial, healthy breakfast soon after rising. According to one study, women who ate larger morning meals consumed fewer total daily calories without even trying than when they ate less at breakfast or skipped it entirely.

Fight disease. Vitamin D, the so-called sunshine vitamin (because it's produced by your skin in response to sunlight), is essential for healthy bones, and it also protects against cardiovascular disease, multiple sclerosis, diabetes, rheumatoid arthritis, and many cancers.

Researchers at Johns Hopkins found that colon cancer deaths were high in New York, New Hampshire, and Vermont, the northern states that get the least amount of daily solar radiation in the continental United States, and low in New Mexico and Arizona, the southern states that get the most. A recent large study found that postmenopausal women who took 1,100 IU of vitamin D along with calcium substantially reduced their risk of all cancers.

Although vitamin D supplements provide some protection against disease, Michael F. Holick, MD, PhD, a professor at the Boston University School of Medicine and author of *The UV Advantage*, believes that short intervals of unprotected sun exposure three times each week confer even more. "I always put sunscreen on my face, which is where most skin cancers occur," says Dr. Holick. "But I leave my arms and legs bare for 15 to 30 minutes before applying it there." In that time, your body can produce 4,000 IU of D, which is the equivalent of 40 glasses of fortified milk.

OUTWIT JET LAG

Why is it that the first thing you want to do on your trip to an exotic locale is nap? Speeding across time zones disrupts the circadian rhythms, resulting in outright exhaustion and, paradoxically, trouble zonking out (or staying zonked). First go-to: Caffeine is a popular and effective pick-me-up, but drinking it after 4 p.m. local time could actually hinder your Zzzs.

Send that fatigue packing by giving these remedies a try.

SEE THE LIGHT. If you're traveling to an earlier time zone, get as much light between 4 and 7 a.m. (home time) by leaving curtains open or touring outdoor sights. If you're traveling to a later time zone, limit light between 4 and 7 a.m. by wearing a sleep mask or sunglasses.

"Learning how to manipulate your exposure to light is important because it governs your internal 24-hour clock, which sets your daily pattern of sleep and wakefulness," says Chris Idzikowsi, PhD, director of the Edinburgh Sleep Centre in Edinburgh, Scotland. "The critical period for adjusting the clock seems to be between 4 and 7 a.m. (home time)."

EAT STRATEGICALLY. Eat lightly the day before you leave. The day of your flight, have a protein-packed breakfast and lunch and a carbohydrate-based dinner. Repeat this routine for your return trip, remembering to again eat lightly the day before your flight.

"Protein-rich foods raise levels of amino acids, which encourage alertness, as opposed to carbohydrates, which stimulate the release of sleep-inducing melatonin," says Ronald D. Novak, PhD, MPH, circadian rhythms expert at Case Western University School of Medicine. "So eat protein in the morning, carbs at night."

You can't overdose on vitamin D from sunshine, but too much sun poses a greater cancer risk to people with fair complexions. To safely ensure you're getting enough daily D, strive for 1,000 IU in food and supplements combined. That's particularly true if you live anywhere north of

Atlanta (33 degrees latitude) in the winter, when the sun is at too low of an angle for you to produce the vitamin. Otherwise, max out your protection against disease by letting the sun shine now and then—on you!

EVENING

Sleep deep in the dark.

Nightfall prompts the release of melatonin, which is a hormone that not only helps bring on drowsiness and sleep but also keeps estrogen levels in check. Without enough melatonin, estrogen rises, which scientists believe might be one of the reasons that female night-shift workers have an increased risk of breast cancer. (In 2007, the World Health Organization classified shift work as a "probable" carcinogen.) Research has also linked the night shift to increases in colorectal and prostate cancers. Follow these habits to ensure proper melatonin levels and reduce your risk of disease.

Forgo bright overhead lights in the evening. Even 30 minutes of exposure to a light slightly brighter than the ones you find in your office can suppress melatonin production. Instead, use task lamps with 40- to 60-watt incandescent bulbs for washing dishes, reading, or watching television or working on the computer.

When sleeping, keep the room as dark as possible. If you use a night-light in your bedroom, equip it with a 7-watt incandescent bulb. It's okay to briefly turn on a low-wattage lightbulb for a bathroom run.

fast fact --
873: The number of Los Angeles County schools cleaned up by Robina Suwol's efforts (See related story on next page.)

HEALTH HEROES

She's keeping school kids safe from dangerous pesticides

One day in 1998, Robina Suwol watched a school gardener spray a stream of pesticides in her son's path. When the weed killer triggered the 6-year-old's asthma, Suwol started digging—and found it contained carcinogens and neurotoxins. Rallying parents and pest-control experts, Suwol, now 52, helped Los Angeles schools adopt a pesticide policy that serves as a model for the nation. In 2006, her organization sponsored a California bill that banned experimental chemicals at all public schools.

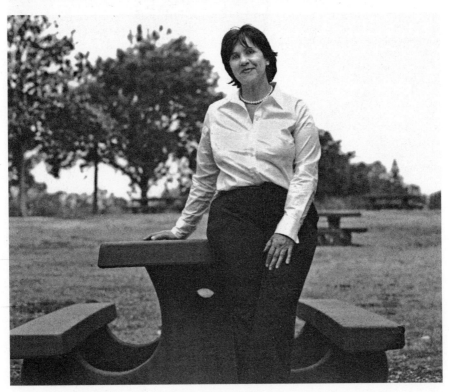

PART

II

NUTRITION NEWS

8

BETTER YOUR DIET

Simple substitutions improve your diet easily—and deliciously

If Americans had a national vegetable, it would probably be french fries. Collectively, our diets could use a lot of improvement.

Fortunately, with some easy substitutions, you could improve your diet—and your health. Take fruit, for example. Although Americans are eating more fruit these days (go us!), more than half are the old standbys: bananas, apples, and oranges. Yes, they're good for you, but you're missing out. "Different fruits provide an array of disease-fighting vitamins, minerals, and antioxidants," says Joy Bauer, RD, author of *Joy Bauer's Food Cures*. In fact, broadening your horizons can measurably improve your health. Colorado State University nutritionists asked 106 women to eat 8 to 10 servings of produce daily for 8 weeks. Half the group chose from 18 different varieties, while the others ate the same 5 over and over again. Two weeks later, blood tests showed that the high-variety group reduced their rates of DNA oxidation, possibly making their bodies more resilient against disease; the other group had no change.

Ready to mix it up? Here's a quickie primer on some of the smartest "exotic" food picks based on their health benefits—and how to serve them in place of common favorites.

FOR PERFECT BLOOD PRESSURE

Good: Bananas

Better: Fresh figs

Why: Six fresh figs have 891 milligrams of blood pressure–lowering potassium, nearly 20 percent of your daily need—about double what you'd find in one large banana. In a recent 5-year study from the Netherlands, high-potassium diets were linked with lower rates of death from all causes in healthy adults age 55 and older.

You'll also get . . . a boost to your bones. Figs are one of the best fruit sources of calcium, with nearly as much per serving (six figs) as ½ cup of fat-free milk!

Shop for figs that are dry on the surface and feel heavy in the hand. A perfectly ripe fig may have slight cracks that are bursting with the fruit's sweet syrup.

Serve by chopping and adding to yogurt, cottage cheese, oatmeal, or green salads. Or enjoy them as a savory snack: Cut a slit in the side and stuff with ½ teaspoon of a low-fat version of a soft cheese such as chèvre or Brie.

TO PROTECT YOUR HEART AND FIGHT DISEASE

Good: Red grapes

Better: Lychee

Why: A French study published in the *Journal of Nutrition* found that lychee has the second-highest level of heart-healthy polyphenols of all fruits tested—nearly 15 percent more than the amount found in grapes, which has been cited by many as a polyphenol powerhouse. The compounds may also play an important role in the prevention of degenerative diseases such as cancer. "Polyphenols act like a force field, helping to repel foreign invaders from damaging your cells," says David Grotto, RD, author of *101 Foods That Could Save Your Life*.

You'll also get . . . protection from breast cancer. A recent test-tube and animal study from Sichuan University in China found that lychee may help prevent the formation of breast cancer cells, thanks to the fruit's powerful antioxidant activity.

Shop for lychee with few black marks on the rough, leathery shell, which can be anywhere from red to brown in color. Look for fruit that gives when pressed gently. Shells should be intact, and the fruit should be attached to the stem.

Serve by peeling or breaking the outer covering just below the stem; use a knife to remove the black pit. Add to stir-fries or skewer onto chicken kebabs to add a sweet, grapelike flavor.

TO LOWER CHOLESTEROL

Good: Apples

Better: Asian pears

Why: One large Asian pear has just about 10 grams of cholesterol-lowering fiber, about 40 percent of your daily need; a large apple has about half that much. People who ate the most fiber had the lowest total and "bad" cholesterol levels, according to a recent study of Baltimore adults.

You'll also get . . . protection from creeping weight gain. The same researchers found that people who ate the most fiber also weighed the least and had the lowest body mass index and waist circumference.

Shop for pears with a firm feel, fragrant aroma, and blemish-free, yellow brownish skin. Some pears are speckled in appearance; the markings shouldn't affect flavor.

Serve by dicing it into a salad of Boston lettuce, crumbled goat cheese, walnuts, and mandarin oranges. Or make it a dessert: Add peeled and cored pears to a saucepan with 1 cup white wine, 1 teaspoon honey, 1 teaspoon grated fresh ginger, and enough water to cover the pears. Cover and simmer for 40 minutes, or until the pears are soft.

TO FIGHT CANCER

Good: Watermelon

Better: Papaya

Why: It is one of the top sources of beta-cryptoxanthin, which research suggests can protect against lung cancer. Like watermelon, it is also a rich source of lycopene. "Although there is currently no recommendation for how much lycopene you should consume in a day, research shows that the nutrient may protect against several different types of cancer, including stomach, endometrial, and prostate," says Grotto.

You'll also get . . . better healing. Papayas may help speed burn recovery when used topically, thanks partly to the enzyme papain, which also aids in digestion. "Papain helps break down amino acids, the building blocks of protein," says Elisa Zied, RD, an American Dietetic Association spokesperson.

Shop for a papaya that has a yellow-golden skin and yields easily to gentle pressure from your grip.

Serve by cutting lengthwise and discarding the black seeds. Scoop out the flesh using a spoon and sprinkle with lemon juice. Or combine chopped papaya, mango, red bell pepper, red onion, raspberries, lemon juice, and cilantro for a fruit salsa. Serve over grilled fish.

FOR BETTER DIGESTION

Good: Yogurt

Better: Kefir

Why: Kefir contains more active cultures than yogurt does. This fermented drink repopulates the army of beneficial bacteria that help fight unwelcome digestive germs. More and more studies are suggesting that cultured foods, such as kefir, protect the intestines, and they also enhance overall immunity.

You'll also get . . . bone-building calcium. An 8-ounce glass of kefir contains 300 milligrams of calcium, which is almost one-third of the recommended daily amount.

Shop for kefir in health food stores and some larger grocery stores. It is available in many fruit flavors.

Serve by sipping it like a smoothie, as a healthy alternative to ice cream, or to replace sour cream or yogurt in recipes. *Note:* People with lactose intolerance will probably have trouble digesting kefir.

FOR BEAUTIFUL SKIN

Good: Orange

Better: Guava

Why: One cup of guava has nearly five times as much skin-healing vitamin C (which is a key ingredient in collagen production) as a medium orange (377 milligrams versus 83 milligrams). That's more than five times your daily need. Women who eat a lot of vitamin C–packed foods have fewer wrinkles than women who don't eat many, according to a recent study that tracked the diets of more than 4,000 American women between the ages of 40 to 74.

You'll also get . . . bacteria-busting power. Guava can protect against food-borne pathogens such as listeria and staph, according to research by microbiologists in Bangladesh. Also, a cooperative study by the USDA and scientists in Thailand found that guava has as much antioxidant activity as some well-known superfoods such as blueberries and broccoli (though every plant contains a different mix of the healthful compounds).

Shop for guava using your nose. A ripe guava has a flowery fragrance, gives a bit to the touch, and has a thin, pale green to light yellowish rind.

Serve by adding to fruit cobbler recipes (the tiny seeds are edible) or simmer chunks in water as you would to make applesauce. Guava also makes a super smoothie: Blend ½ banana, ½ ripe guava, a handful of strawberries, ½ cup soy milk, and a few ice cubes. To ripen a guava, put it in a brown paper bag with a banana. Leave it out at room temperature until the guava begins to soften.

FOR STRONG MUSCLES

Good: Couscous

Better: Quinoa

Why: Although couscous provides a healthy supply of protein to build muscles, quinoa has an almost perfect balance of amino acids, which makes it a superior source of protein. It contains all eight amino acids that muscles need to grow, and it is especially high in lysine, which is an essential acid the body uses for tissue repair.

You'll also get . . . healthy unsaturated fats. Unlike many high-protein foods, quinoa is low in saturated fats and high in unsaturated ones.

Shop for quinoa in a variety of colors, including orange, purple, and pink. The most commonly available is a transparent yellow color. You can find packaged quinoa in most health food stores or grocery stores. Quinoa cereal, crackers, cookies, flour, and bread are also available. The seeds should be sealed in a plastic or glass container and stored in a cool, dry area. Moisture and sunlight can cause the oils to go rancid.

Serve by making your own quinoa cereal: Cook it in orange juice and serve it with honey and pecans. Or cook it with cubed butternut squash for a hearty winter porridge. Be sure to rinse quinoa in cool water before cooking it. Quinoa is naturally coated in saponin, which is a bitter-tasting substance that can cause indigestion.

fast fact ---

88: The percentage of children ages 11 to 15 who do not eat the recommended five-a-day fruits and veggies (See related story on next page.)

HEALTH HEROES

Their campaign aims to fix 27 million school lunches a day

Susan Rubin's crusade began with the candy wrappers in her first-grader's backpack. The Chappaqua, New York, dentist and nutritionist, 46, joined Weston, Connecticut, filmmaker Amy Kalafa to expose horrors in America's cafeterias, including trans fat–filled snacks and lunches without vegetables.

"Eliminating bad food is a start," says Kalafa, 48, "but districts need help finding fresh, tasty options, too." Their documentary, *Two Angry Moms*, aims to recruit 2 million moms to fight for healthy school menus.

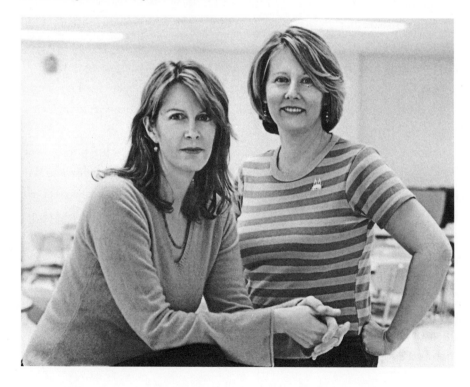

DOUBLE YOUR NUTRITION

Nine ways to chop, sauté, and stir your way to better health

Stocked up on leafy greens? Super. Did you know that sautéing them in a bit of olive oil instead of steaming them will help you absorb up to five times as much of the vision-protecting antioxidant beta-carotene? Buying healthy food is just the first step toward a better diet; preparing it correctly can make or break your nutrient bank. Keep reading for even more surprising nutrition-enhancing prep tips.

FIRE UP HEART PROTECTION

Heating lycopene-rich tomatoes instigates a chemical change that makes the heart-healthy nutrient much easier for your body to absorb. Try halving Roma tomatoes lengthwise, arrange on a baking sheet, drizzle with olive oil, and season with salt and pepper. Broil for 15 to 20 minutes, until slightly shriveled. Adding canned crushed tomatoes or tomato paste to recipes works, too. They were heated during processing.

MAXIMIZE CANCER PREVENTION

High temperatures will destroy allinase, garlic's most important cancer-fighting and immunity-boosting enzyme. After chopping, let crushed garlic stand for 10 to 15 minutes before adding it to a sizzling pan. This allows the pungent herb to generate compounds that blunt the damaging effects of heat, report scientists at Pennsylvania State University and the National Cancer Institute.

No time to spare? You can always enjoy raw garlic. We love rubbing it on toasted bread and topping it with chopped tomato and onion and a dash of olive oil for a simple bruschetta.

GET 10 TIMES THE IRON

Cooking with tomatoes, apples, or lemons? Heat acidic foods such as these in a cast-iron pot or skillet to spike the amount of the energy-boosting iron you absorb by more than 2,000 percent, suggests a Texas Tech University study.

"Some iron from the skillet leaches into the food, but the particles are small enough that you won't be able to see or taste them, and it's perfectly safe," says Cynthia Sass, RD, MPH, *Prevention*'s nutrition director.

Bonus tip: You don't have to pull out a pan; coupling certain iron-rich foods with high-acid ones gives a tenfold boost to your iron absorption. "While the iron in red meat is easily absorbed on its own, the type of iron found in beans, grains, and veggies isn't," Sass says. When making a spinach salad, toss in mango slices to increase the iron payoff. Other healthy combos: beans and tomato sauce or cereal and strawberries.

STRENGTHEN EYES AND BONES

Adding avocado, olive oil, nuts, olives, or another healthy fat source to red, green, orange, and yellow fruits and veggies increases the amount of fat-soluble vitamins, such as A, E, and K. These nutrients boost vision, improve immunity, and protect against stroke and osteoporosis, respectively.

"Fat acts as a transporter for them," explains Sass. The same strategy works for carotenoids, the compounds that give tomatoes and carrots their bright hues. Proof: A recent study from the Ohio State University Comprehensive Cancer Center found that men and women who ate salsa containing chunks of avocado absorbed 4.4 times as much lycopene and 2.6 times as much beta-carotene than those who enjoyed plain salsa.

STOCK UP ON CALCIUM

If you're preparing homemade chicken soup, it's smart to add a hint of lemon juice, vinegar, or tomato to the mix. Pairing a slightly acidic broth with on-the-bone chicken can up the soup's calcium content by 64 percent, according to researchers at Harvard University and Beth Israel Hospital in Boston. This stock dissolves the bone's calcium more easily than a nonacidic one would.

Bonus tip: Other research that was referenced in the Harvard/Beth Israel study has shown that slathering spareribs with an acidic vinegar-based barbecue sauce will dramatically increase the calcium content.

GRILL WITHOUT WORRY

The high heat needed to grill meats can create carcinogenic compounds called heterocyclic amines (HCAs), but marinating can help. When researchers at Lawrence Livermore National Laboratory in Livermore, California, soaked chicken breasts in a mixture of brown sugar, olive oil, cider vinegar, garlic, mustard, lemon juice, and salt for 4 hours, they developed up to 99 percent fewer HCAs after 20 minutes of grilling than unmarinated chicken did.

Try that marinade, or add an extra antioxidant kick with this herb-packed soak: ½ cup of balsamic vinegar; 2 tablespoons of fresh rosemary; 1 tablespoon each of olive oil, honey, and minced garlic; and ½ teaspoon of ground black pepper.

Bonus tip: Instead of marinating hamburgers (too messy), mix in some rosemary. Research has found that it can slash the production of some HCAs by as much as 72 percent.

FIGHT COLDS AND FLU

When you're slicing fresh produce, cut large pieces. Smaller portions expose more of the fruit or vegetable to nutrient-leaching oxygen and light.

"A larger cut allows you to hold on to more vitamin C, which helps bolster immunity," says Roberta Larson Duyff, RD, author of the *American Dietetic Association Complete Food and Nutrition Guide*. Quarter carrots, potatoes, and tomatoes instead of dicing them; slice melons into crescents rather than cubing.

RETAIN KEY NUTRIENTS

Save yourself some time—and some key nutrients—by not peeling eggplant, apples, potatoes, and other produce before using.

"The peel itself is a natural barrier against nutrient loss, and many vitamins and minerals are found in the outer skin or just below it," Duyff says. Yam skin is loaded with fiber, and zucchini's is full of lutein, which may help prevent age-related macular degeneration, for example. Remove grit and pathogens with cold, running water and a vegetable brush.

Bonus tip: Add citrus zest to your favorite recipes. A University of Arizona study linked eating limonene, which is a compound in lemon, lime, and orange peel, to a 34 percent reduction in skin cancer.

DOUBLE THE ANTIOXIDANTS

Dressing your salad with herbs can more than double its cancer-fighting punch, according to a recent Italian study. When compared with garden salads made with no added herbs, those featuring lemon balm and marjoram had up to 200 percent more antioxidants per serving. Spices such as ginger and cumin also upped the antioxidant quotient.

CHAPTER 10

COOK LIKE YOUR LIFE DEPENDS ON IT!

Make these small changes in the way you prepare food and transform your meals into nutritional superstars

Piling your shopping cart high with healthful staples such as veggies, fish, and lean meat? Great! Now, take it to the next level. It's what you do with those fantastic foods once you bring them home that can promote them to the real nutritional diva level. Take the tomato: Eat it cooked instead of raw and you'll get as much as 171 percent more of the cancer-fighting compound lycopene. "Even one little change in the kitchen can result in a huge health payoff," says Robin Plotkin, RD, a Dallas-based nutritionist. Follow our simple rules for cooking smarter and amp up the disease-fighting power of every meal. Then try the delicious sample recipes that follow.

BAKE TOMATOES

For: Younger skin (and cancer protection)

Compared with fresh tomatoes, cooked tomatoes (and products such as pasta sauce) contain more lycopene, which is a powerful antioxidant. Research suggests that lycopene may guard the skin against damage from the sun's UV rays. Baking tomatoes makes them healthier and more versatile, adding a flavorful twist to sandwiches, salads, and pastas.

How: Wash and pat dry 30 cherry or grape tomatoes. Place them in a small baking dish and drizzle them with 1 tablespoon olive oil. Bake at 450°F for 15 minutes.

BAKED TOMATO, MOZZARELLA, AND ROASTED TURKEY SANDWICHES

2 SERVINGS ■ 223 CALORIES

1 small whole wheat baguette

½ teaspoon Dijon mustard

2 ounces sliced roasted turkey breast

2 ounces reduced-fat sliced mozzarella cheese

15 hot, baked cherry tomatoes

1. HALVE the baguette lengthwise and spread Dijon mustard on the lower half.

2. LAYER on the roasted turkey breast, mozzarella cheese, and cherry tomatoes.

3. COVER with the top baguette portion and slice in half.

NUTRITION PER SERVING

223 calories, 19 g protein, 21 g carbohydrates, 7 g fat, 4 g saturated fat, 35 mg cholesterol, 353 mg sodium, 3 g fiber

KITCHEN CURE

Store watermelon at room temperature. Leaving a whole watermelon on your kitchen counter for 5 days increases its lycopene and beta-carotene content by as much as 20 percent.

ROAST OMEGA-3–RICH FISH

For: A slimmer waistline

Roasting a fatty fish, such as salmon, with a bit of olive oil doesn't increase its fat content, according to a study published in the *Journal of Agriculture and Food Chemistry*. When researchers fried the fish, it absorbed the olive oil, increasing fat content by about 10 percent (and adding unnecessary calories).

How: Drizzle baking dish with olive oil. Select fresh fish fillets, approximately ⅓ pound per person. Roast fish skin side down in a dish in a 450°F oven until a meat thermometer reaches an internal temperature of 145°F degrees, or 10 minutes per inch of thickness. Properly prepared fish will flake easily with a fork. (Overcooking makes it dry.) Remove from oven; serve immediately.

ROASTED FISH FILLETS

2 SERVINGS ■ 241 CALORIES

1 teaspoon olive oil

2 5-ounce fish fillets, such as salmon or lake trout

Juice from 1 small lemon

1 clove garlic, crushed

⅛ teaspoon ground pepper

¼ cup fresh parsley

1. PREHEAT the oven to 450°F.

2. LIGHTLY coat a small baking dish with oil and place the fish fillets in the dish.

3. SPRINKLE with the lemon juice, garlic, and pepper.

4. ROAST for 10 minutes per inch of thickness.

5. SPRINKLE with the parsley.

NUTRITION PER SERVING

241 calories, 30 g protein, 3 g carbohydrates, 12 g fat, 2 g saturated fat, 82 mg cholesterol, 78 mg sodium, 0.5 g fiber

Serving suggestion: Serve with a grain of your choice, such as quinoa or wild rice, and steamed veggies.

CRUSH GARLIC

For: Healthier arteries

Crushing garlic cloves—and letting them stand for 10–15 minutes before heating them—activates and preserves the heart-protecting compounds in the garlic, according to a study from Argentina. Cooking uncrushed garlic for as little as 6 minutes can completely suppress its protective strength.

How: Wash and peel the outer papery skins of a clove of garlic and trim the ends. To crush, place the clove on a cutting board and lay the flat side of a wide knife against it, pressing down firmly. For easier use in recipes, finely chop the clove, starting at one side. Crush again: Press the flat side of the knife against the chopped garlic firmly, then finely chop again. Let it rest for 30 minutes at room temperature. Scrape the crushed and chopped pieces and juice from the cutting board into the recipe.

GARLIC BEAN CHOWDER

6 SERVINGS ■ 81 CALORIES

1 teaspoon extra virgin olive oil

1 cup chopped onion

1 cup chopped celery

1 cup chopped carrots

4 cloves garlic, crushed and chopped

2½ cups low-sodium vegetable broth

1 can (15 ounces) cannellini beans, with liquid

2 teaspoons fresh basil

1 teaspoon freshly squeezed lemon juice

1 bay leaf

¼ teaspoon freshly ground black pepper

1. HEAT the oil in a large, heavy pot.

2. ADD the onion, celery, carrots, and garlic and sauté for 2 minutes.

3. ADD the broth, beans, basil, lemon juice, bay leaf, and pepper.

4. COVER and simmer for 25 to 30 minutes over medium heat.

5. REMOVE the bay leaf.

NUTRITION PER SERVING

81 calories, 15 g protein, 1 g carbohydrates, 1 g fat, 0 g saturated fat, 0 mg cholesterol, 201 mg sodium, 4 g fiber

Serving suggestion: Serve with salad and whole-grain flatbread.

STEAM BROCCOLI

For: Reduced cancer risk

Steaming broccoli increases its content of glucosinolates, which are compounds that fight cancer. Other cooking techniques, such as frying, reduce them, according to new research from Parma, Italy.

How: Clean and trim 1 pound of broccoli, cutting into florets. Bring 1 inch of water to a boil in a saucepan. Place the florets in a metal colander over the boiling water. Cover and reduce the heat to medium. Cook until tender, about 6 to 7 minutes. (Or you can microwave on high in a covered but vented dish for that time.)

STIR-FRIED SHRIMP AND STEAMED BROCCOLI

4 SERVINGS ■ 238 CALORIES

1 teaspoon vegetable oil

1 pound shrimp, peeled and deveined

1 tablespoon reduced-sodium soy sauce

1 clove garlic, crushed

1 teaspoon minced ginger

⅛ teaspoon ground white pepper

1 teaspoon red curry paste

1 pound broccoli, cut into florets and steamed

½ cup reduced-sodium chicken broth

1 teaspoon cornstarch

⅓ cup dry-roasted unsalted cashews

1. HEAT the oil in a large skillet.

2. ADD the shrimp, soy sauce, garlic, ginger, pepper, and curry paste. Sauté for 2 minutes. Stir in the broccoli.

3. WHISK together the broth and cornstarch in a small bowl. Add to the skillet and stir until thick.

4. REMOVE from the heat; the shrimp should be opaque.

5. GARNISH with the cashews.

NUTRITION PER SERVING

238 calories, 29 g protein, 12 g carbohydrates, 9 g fat, 1.7 g saturated fat, 172 mg cholesterol, 469 mg sodium, 4 g fiber

SLOW-COOK MEAT

For: Preventing inflammation linked to diabetes and heart disease

When meats are cooked in liquid at moderate heat, they develop fewer cell-damaging compounds known as AGEs (advanced glycation end products) than when they are broiled or grilled. Researchers say that switching to "wet" cooking methods can reduce AGE intake by 50 percent.

How: Trim visible fat from 1 pound of sectioned beef, pork, or poultry. Place in a slow cooker. Add 1 cup of liquid (such as broth). Add vegetables and seasonings. Cover and cook on high for 1 hour. Reduce to low and cook for 2 to 8 hours longer (depending on the thickness and type of meat), until the meat reaches an internal temperature of 145°F for beef, 160°F for pork, and 165°F for poultry.

MANGO GINGER CHICKEN

4 SERVINGS ■ 209 CALORIES

1 pound chicken breast tenderloins

2 carrots, sliced

2 ribs celery, chopped

1 onion, sliced

1 cup frozen peas

1 cup mango nectar

2 cloves garlic, crushed

1½ teaspoons freshly crushed ginger

1 teaspoon ground white pepper

1 teaspoon reduced-sodium soy sauce

½ teaspoon ground turmeric

2 teaspoons cornstarch

1. PLACE the chicken breast tenderloins, carrots, celery, onion, peas, mango nectar, garlic, ginger, pepper, soy sauce, and turmeric in a slow cooker.

2. COVER and cook for 1 hour on high.

3. REDUCE the heat to low and cook for 2 hours longer.

4. REMOVE ½ cup of liquid to a small bowl, stir in the cornstarch, and then add back to the slow cooker.

5. COVER and cook on low for 1 hour longer.

NUTRITION PER SERVING

209 calories, 29 g protein, 24 g carbohydrates, 1 g fat, 0 g saturated fat, 67 mg cholesterol, 186 mg sodium, 4 g fiber

Serving suggestion: Serve with brown rice.

TRY THE NEW SUPERFOODS

Move over, blueberries. There's a new pack of disease-fighting vittles in town

Had it up to here with broccoli? Join the club. But it's hard to take it off the menu when it's such a great source of vitamins and minerals. Still, is a little variety too much to ask?

Not anymore, thanks to research that's shifting the spotlight to a new generation of health-boosting foods—many of which do double or triple duty to help prevent illness. Here are six on the brink of superstar status.

POMEGRANATE

If you're going to have a martini, at least make it a pomegranate one. This fall fruit has higher antioxidant activity than red wine and green tea, which may be why a number of studies show it may prevent skin cancer and kill breast and prostate cancer cells. It also helps in the following ways.

Fight Alzheimer's disease. Researchers at Loma Linda University found that mice who drank pomegranate juice experienced 50 percent less brain degeneration than animals that consumed only sugar water. The pomegranate drinkers also did better in mazes and tests as they aged.

Guard your arteries. A group of people with diabetes who drank about 2 ounces of pomegranate juice a day for 3 months kept their bodies from absorbing bad cholesterol into their immune system cells, which is a major contributing factor to hardened arteries, discovered Israeli researchers.

KIWIFRUIT

Don't judge this fruit by its cover: Under that bristly brown peel you'll find a bright green star bursting with antioxidants and fiber. Kiwifruit works to help in the following ways.

Protect against free radical damage. A study from Rutgers University compared the 27 most popular fruits and determined that kiwifruit was the most nutritionally dense. Plus, it makes the short list of fruits with substantial amounts of vitamin E, and contains more vision-saving lutein than any other fruit or vegetable, except for corn.

Lower blood clot risk. In a 2004 study from the University of Oslo in Norway, participants who ate two or three kiwis for 28 days significantly reduced their potential to form a clot. They also got a bonus benefit: Their triglycerides, a blood fat linked to heart attack, dropped by 15 percent.

BARLEY

When some whole grains, such as wheat and oats, are processed, they lose their fiber content. Not so with barley, which is full of soluble beta-glucan fiber in its whole kernel or refined flour form. Studies show this particular fiber may offer the following benefits.

Knock down bad cholesterol. Barley lowers the bad kind by as much as 17.4 percent, according to USDA research. A 2004 study found that adults with moderately high cholesterol levels who went on a low-fat

HEALTHIER FOOD HUES

More than just novelties, these three fruits and veggies have been bred to be better for you.

Orange Cauliflower

ORIGIN: Developed from a mutant strain by a Cornell University researcher.

BONUS: Contains 25 times more vitamin A than its white sibling.

BetaSweet Carrot

ORIGIN: A Texas A&M scientist gave this vegetable a maroon coat to match the school's colors.

BONUS: Rich in antioxidants, it offers 40 percent more beta-carotene than regular carrots.

Black Krim Tomato

ORIGIN: Part of a crop category called heirloom tomatoes, this deep reddish brown fruit hails from Russia.

BONUS: Its spicy and slightly salty flavor tastes great, and it's a good source of lycopene and vitamin C.

American Heart Association diet began to see an improvement only when barley was added to the menu.

Decrease blood sugar and insulin levels. That makes barley a better choice for people with type 2 diabetes, says a 2005 Agricultural Research Services study.

CRANBERRY

This born-and-bred American berry is among the top 10 antioxidant-rich foods, making it a potent cancer protector. You know that it helps

(continued on page 100)

POWER FOODS FOR FITNESS

Taking up a new exercise program? The key to a better workout—and a bigger calorie burn—is eating nutrient-dense foods about 30 minutes before you start exercising. For starters, try these picks from Tara Gidus, RD, a sports dietitian based in Orlando. They're all packed with high-quality carbohydrates, which provide a quick source of fuel for your muscles, but they have just enough protein and fat to help you maintain a steady, elevated energy level. To maximize the weight-loss benefits of exercise, keep calories to about 200 or less.

Apples

One a day may keep the doctor away, but three a day may help you drop pounds, according to research from the University of Rio de Janeiro in Brazil. More important, apples are exceptionally high in antioxidants, which can help offset the damage caused by free radicals, an unfortunate by-product of daily exercise. The perfect protein/fat addition? Natural unsweetened nut butters. Just spread them on sparingly to keep calories under control.

TRY: A sliced apple with 2 teaspoons of peanut or almond butter (150 calories).

Chicken Soup

It's quick, easy, and can help you lose weight, according to research from Pennsylvania State University. But soup can also keep you hydrated during your walk. Look for low-sodium options that provide lean protein (such as chicken breast), vegetables (for antioxidants), and a source of carbohydrates (such as rice or noodles).

TRY: Progresso 50% Less Sodium Chicken Gumbo (220 calories per can).

Trail Mix

You don't need an expensive mix loaded with candy-coated whatnot. An excellent trail mix for walkers is a handful each of nuts (walnuts are high in anti-inflammatory omega-3 fatty acids) and raisins (which offer a concentrated source of energy).

TRY: Eight walnut halves plus a mini box (0.5 ounce) of raisins (150 calories).

Nutrition Bars

The right one supplies about twice as much carbohydrates as protein and about 5 grams of fat and 3 grams of fiber. Oh, and it shouldn't taste like cardboard.

TRY: Luna Bar Caramel Nut Brownie flavor (190 calories).

Yogurt

Most yogurts offer an ideal activity-fueling protein-carb combination, but pick one that's unsweetened; sugar-laden fruit flavorings add unnecessary calories without the fiber of whole fruit. (Bonus benefit: Eating three daily servings of dairy foods such as yogurt provides bone-building calcium, which also helps muscles contract.)

TRY: Low-fat plain yogurt with ½ cup of chopped fruit or berries (175 calories).

Chocolate Milk

After a workout, your muscles need protein to repair microscopic muscle tears, plus another shot of carbs to help restock energy stores. In an Indiana University study, cyclists who drank reduced-fat chocolate milk after a tough racing session had improved endurance and recovered faster than those who drank an ordinary sports drink (which supplies carbs and electrolytes, but no protein).

Try: 8 ounces of reduced-fat chocolate milk (190 calories).

treat urinary tract infection, and perhaps you heard it prevents gum disease, too. But did you know that these beneficial berries may do the following for you as well?

Eradicate *Escherichia coli*. Compounds that are in the juice can actually alter antibiotic-resistant strains, making it impossible for the harmful bacteria to trigger an infection. Likewise, a small pilot study conducted at the Harvard Medical School and Rutgers University found that just eating about ⅓ cup of dried cranberries similarly yielded the same effect.

Help prevent strokes. During research performed on pigs with a genetic predisposition to atherosclerosis—narrow, hardened arteries that may lead to heart attack and stroke—it was discovered that those pigs fed dried cranberries or cranberry juice every day had healthier, more flexible blood vessels.

BROCCOLI SPROUTS

Yes, we've been through this—broccoli, good. The news: Broccoli sprouts are even better. At a mere 3 days old, they contain at least 20 times as much of disease-fighting sulforaphane glucosinolate (SGS) as their elders; SGS has been shown to have these benefits.

Kill tumors. The chemical triggers enzymes in the body that either kill cancer cells or keep them from growing. Just 1 ounce of these potent sprouts has as much SGS as 1¼ pounds of broccoli plus that will even save you lots of chewing.

Protect your heart. People who ate about a half cup a day of sprouts lowered their total cholesterol by an average of 15 points, and women in the study raised their good cholesterol by 8 points—in just 1 week, found a Japanese pilot study.

Save your sight. Exposure to harmful UV sunlight over time can possibly lead to an eye condition called macular degeneration, which is the number one cause of blindness in US seniors. Researchers at Johns Hopkins determined that broccoli sprouts can protect the retinal cells from ultraviolet light damage.

KEFIR

We already extolled the virtues of kefir in chapter 8, but we think it warrants more praise here. This cultured milk drink stacks up in calcium—one 8-ounce serving contains 30 percent of the recommended daily intake, and it also contains more beneficial bacteria than yogurt. It may also do the following.

Reduce food allergies. Baby mice fed kefir had a threefold reduction in the amount of an antibody linked to food allergies, say researchers at an agricultural university.

Battle breast cancer. Women age 50 and older who consumed fermented milk products had a lower risk of breast cancer than those who ate little or none.

Avoid triggering lactose intolerance. Kefir contains lactase, the enzyme that people with lactose intolerance are missing, say researchers at Ohio State University. (Though other researchers say kefir can trigger lactose intolerance in some people.) And the taste? Like plain yogurt, just a little thinner.

CHAPTER 12

EAT FOR ALL-DAY ENERGY

You can beat fatigue by eating
the right foods. Feel better fast
with these tailor-made menus

Quick: Name your usual tiredness fix. If you said a cereal bar or a coffee drink, you're not getting an effective boost, and you may even be setting yourself up to crash later on. "The food you eat is like the gas you use to fuel your car," says Bonnie Taub-Dix, RD, a spokesperson for the American Dietetic Association. "Without enough of it—or the right kind—your energy will stall." Luckily, certain foods can help fight fatigue.

Here are some of the top stamina sappers you may encounter, and what to eat and drink more of (sample menus included!) to stay sharp, focused, and energized all day.

ENERGY SAPPER: STRESS

Tension, whether it's caused by your job, kids, or caring for aging parents, triggers a surge in hormones such as cortisol and adrenaline, which can lead to fatigue and related symptoms like headache and back pain. A stressful lifestyle may also leave you with little time to prepare energizing, healthful meals.

Eat More

Carb-rich foods: Healthy treats such as half of a whole wheat English muffin with fruit spread are rich in carbohydrates, which can boost your levels of serotonin, a calming brain chemical.

Chocolate: Nibbling on a few squares of dark chocolate may work, too. It's packed with caffeine and theobromine, which are mild mood- and energy-boosting stimulants, according to UK researchers.

Fluid-filled foods: "Food accounts for about 20 percent of our daily fluid intake," says Samuel N. Cheuvront, PhD, RD, a principal investigator with the US Army Research Institute of Environmental Medicine. Staying hydrated is one of the simplest ways to keep energized and focused. A recent study of athletes found that 92 percent felt fatigued after limiting fluids and water-rich foods for 15 hours; they also had lapses in memory and reported difficulty concentrating.

To eat for energy, avoid dry packaged snacks such as pretzels, which lack sufficient fluid to aid hydration. Instead, opt for water-rich snacks, including fresh produce. Foods that swell up during cooking—such as oatmeal and pasta (which is nearly 65 percent water)—are also smart choices.

Drink More

Tea: A recent report found that pairing caffeine and the amino acid L-theanine, both present in tea, decreased mental fatigue and improved alertness, reaction time, and memory. What's more, black tea varieties can help you recover from stress, according to researchers at University College London. In the study, adults who drank tea four times a day for

6 weeks had lower levels of the stress hormone cortisol after a tense moment, compared with those who drank a tealike placebo.

Your Stress-Busting Menu

Try these foods to keep your stress at bay.

Breakfast: 1 cup oatmeal made with fat-free milk, topped with 1 diced pear, 2 tablespoons chopped walnuts, and 2 teaspoons brown sugar; 1 cup black tea

Lunch: 1 cup reduced-sodium minestrone soup; ¼ cup hummus with 10 baby carrots, 1 cup cucumber and red bell pepper slices; 2 cups air-popped popcorn

Snack: 2 tablespoons semisweet chocolate chips; 1 cup black tea

Dinner: Spicy Shrimp Spaghetti: 10 large shrimp sautéed in 2 teaspoons olive oil with 1 clove minced garlic and a pinch of red-pepper flakes, tossed with 1 chopped tomato and 1 cup cooked whole grain spaghetti; small salad with 1 tablespoon vinaigrette; 1 orange

Snack: ¾ cup raspberry sorbet

Nutrition information: 1,560 calories, 57 g protein, 248 g carbohydrates, 44 g fat, 10 g saturated fat, 110 mg cholesterol, 840 mg sodium, 38 g fiber

ENERGY SAPPER: DIETING

Calories are literally units of energy. Without the proper amount of fuel your cells need to perform, you'll feel weak and lightheaded. Your challenge: Trim enough calories to lose weight but get the right number to keep energized. Visit Prevention.com/healthtrackers to determine your daily caloric needs, and then follow our smart strategies for slimming down without slowing down.

Eat More

Frequent meals: Small, regular meals and snacks (instead of a few large ones) every 3 to 4 hours give you sustained energy and dampen hunger by keeping your blood sugar on an even keel. When researchers at the National Institute on Aging compared middle-age men and women who ate only one meal a day with those who consumed three squares, they found that the one-meal-a-day group had larger spikes in blood sugar. As a result, eating less frequently may cause energy levels to soar and then plummet.

Fiber: Roughage-rich foods slow digestion, keeping energy stable. They also help fill you up, so you eat less. Choosing foods such as onions, bananas, and whole wheat may help you keep up your stamina and control your weight because they are rich in inulin, a prebiotic fiber, which means it encourages the growth of healthy bacteria in the gut. The substance may keep unwanted pounds at bay by regulating some of the hormones that control appetite, according to researchers at the USDA/ARS Children's Nutrition Research Center in Houston. Right now there's no recommended intake of prebiotic fiber specifically, but getting small amounts throughout the day is a strategy that can help you meet your daily 25 grams of total fiber and drop pounds.

Drink More

Water and unsweetened beverages: Staying hydrated will keep you energized and may help you shed weight. Even mild dehydration can slow metabolism, according to researchers at the University of Utah.

Just avoid artificially sweetened beverages. Although they contribute few calories, a Purdue University study revealed that artificial sweeteners may interfere with your brain's signals, prompting you to eat more. If you don't like water, try another energy-revving drink that will hydrate you without increasing your appetite or adding excess calories, such as tea or sparkling water—either au naturel or flavored with homemade frozen 100 percent fruit juice cubes.

Your Diet-Friendly Menu

Try this menu to keep your calories down but your energy up.

Breakfast: 1 slice whole wheat bread, toasted and topped with 1 tablespoon almond butter and 1 small sliced banana; coffee or tea

Snack: ½ cup fat-free vanilla yogurt with 2 tablespoons dried cranberries; 1 glass of water with lemon

Lunch: Greek Tuna Wrap: 1 cup romaine lettuce tossed with 3 ounces drained chunk light tuna, ½ sliced tomato, 5 black olives, ¼ sliced cucumber, sliced onions, 1 tablespoon red wine vinegar, and 1 teaspoon olive oil, wrapped in 1 whole wheat tortilla; 1 glass of sparkling water with 2 100 percent grape juice ice cubes

Snack: 1 apple; 2 1-inch cubes low-fat cheese; 12 ounces unsweetened iced tea

Dinner: Onion-Smothered Barbecued Chicken: 4 ounces grilled chicken breast with 1 tablespoon barbecue sauce, topped with ½ grilled, sliced onion; 1 baked sweet potato; 6 steamed asparagus spears with 1 teaspoon olive oil

Snack: 2 cups air-popped popcorn sprinkled with 1 teaspoon grated Parmesan cheese; 1 medium orange

Nutrition information: 1,380 calories, 85 g protein, 208 g carbohydrates, 29 g total fat, 5 g saturated fat, 130 mg cholesterol, 1,550 mg sodium, 27 g fiber

ENERGY SAPPER: SLEEP DEPRIVATION

When you're tired, you may feel hungrier than usual. That's because lack of slumber disrupts hormones that signal your need for nourishment.

Eating the right foods can help boost your energy and keep you satisfied without overeating.

Eat More

Sleep-promoting nutrients: "Certain vitamins and minerals have a profound effect on the quality of our slumber," says Elizabeth Somer, RD, author of *Food & Mood*. "Getting adequate amounts of vitamins B_6 and B_{12}, calcium, iron, and magnesium can help you maintain healthy sleep patterns."

One key player is vitamin B_{12}, which we don't absorb as well as we age. The nutrient helps fight fatigue by building strong, healthy red blood cells. Several studies reveal that vitamin B_{12} may improve chronic insomnia by influencing melatonin, a hormone that regulates sleep cycles. Because B_{12} is found only in animal foods, such as turkey and milk, vegetarians and vegans may need to eat fortified foods or take a supplement.

Carbs at night: Before you turn in, try a small bowl of oatmeal or a handful of whole grain crackers for their comforting carbohydrates. An all-carb snack increases levels of mood-lifting serotonin, which may help promote sleep.

Drink More

Small doses of caffeine: Frequent mini-servings of caffeine (8 ounces of coffee or less) keep you awake, alert, and focused for longer than a single jumbo one would, according to sleep experts. "When you quickly drink a large coffee, the caffeine peaks in your bloodstream much sooner than if you spread it out over time," says Harris R. Lieberman, PhD, a research psychologist with the US Army Research Institute of Environmental Medicine.

Start your day with an 8-ounce coffee (the "short" size is available by request at Starbucks). Or ask for a large half caf. Then keep the caffeine lightly flowing with a lunchtime cappuccino (it has only 75 milligrams—about one-quarter of what you'd get in a 16-ounce coffee), followed by a small midafternoon latte. If you have trouble sleeping, you may want to avoid caffeine in the afternoon, or altogether. Not a java junkie? Tea works, too, though it is lower in caffeine.

Your Sleep-Deeply Menu

Try this menu during the day to get more restful sleep at night.

Breakfast: Morning Burrito: 3 egg whites scrambled in 1 teaspoon canola oil with 1 tablespoon shredded low-fat cheese and 2 tablespoons salsa, in a whole wheat tortilla; ½ grapefruit; 8 ounces coffee or 16 ounces half caf

Lunch: Turkey burger on a whole wheat bun with ¼ sliced avocado and sliced tomato and onion; 1 cup grapes; 4 dried apricots; 8 ounces fat-free cappuccino

Snack: 8 ounces fat-free latte; 2 tablespoons nuts with ¼ cup whole grain cereal

Dinner: 3 ounces grilled or broiled lean flank steak; 1 baked potato with 2 tablespoons low-fat plain yogurt and 1 tablespoon chopped chives; 1 cup spinach sautéed in 1 teaspoon olive oil with ½ clove minced garlic

Snack: 1 packet prepared instant oatmeal

Nutrition information: 1,560 calories, 99 g protein, 229 g carbohydrates, 33 g total fat, 6 g saturated fat, 95 mg cholesterol, 1,060 mg sodium, 29 g fiber

IS YOUR MATTRESS KEEPING YOU UP?

Researchers at the Back Research Center in Denmark discovered that women who slept for 1 month on either a water bed or a body-conforming foam mattress got more sleep and had less back pain than those using a firm, spring-free futon.

If you're in the market for a mattress, test it properly to make sure it won't keep you up at night. The mattress should mold to the contours of your neck, back, waist, and knees, while keeping your spine in a neutral position.

CHAPTER 13

GO ORGANIC— WITHOUT GOING BROKE

You can make wholesome choices without spending a lot of green. Here's how

With all the news about rising food costs, you may be wondering whether the organic milk you've been putting in your cart is worth the extra cash. It is. Organic food is more expensive, but when it comes to the staples of your diet, organics are a worthwhile investment, with payoffs that might surprise you. The benefits influence your health today—and long-term. Here, discover why certain foods are worth the cost, plus tips to save you money while keeping your diet nutritionally and ecologically sound.

They have more nutrients. Reports of organic food not being better for you are outdated. A brand-new analysis of about 100 studies, including more than 40 published in the past 7 years, found that the average levels of nearly a dozen nutrients are 25 percent higher in organic produce.

ORGANICS TO SKIP

Step into any health food store and you're likely to find an organic version of just about everything, including cotton candy. Although it's true that organic "junk foods" are better for the planet, they generally aren't better for you. A six-pack of organic soda costs $5; yes, it's made without high-fructose corn syrup, but each can contains 160 calories (20 more than a 12-ounce can of Coca-Cola Classic) and zero nutrients. Cutting back on sweets and nutritionally void extras altogether is the best way to get the most nutrition bang for your buck.

There may be weight benefits. Research in rats found that those fed an all-organic diet (versus conventional food) had lower weights, less body fat, and stronger immune systems. Plus, the "clean diet" animals were calmer and slept better.

You consume fewer toxins. Eating the 12 most contaminated fruits and vegetables exposes you to about 14 pesticides a day. A study supported by the Environmental Protection Agency measured pesticide levels in children's urine before and after a switch to an organic diet. After just 5 days, the chemicals decreased to undetectable levels.

The number one barrier that prevents shoppers from taking advantage of these benefits: cost. Fortunately, you can save on green groceries. Before you purchase any organic food, consider the following cost-saving ideas.

Go generic. Nearly every mainstream supermarket now carries organic store-brand options, including Safeway's O Organics line, H-E-B's Central Market Organic selections, Wal-Mart's Great Value private label, Stop & Shop's Nature's Promise, and SuperValu's Wild Harvest. Organics are also available within Kroger, Publix, and Wegmans store brands.

Join a price club. Organic options can be found at Costco, BJ's, and Sam's Club.

Buy in bulk. You can purchase many organic grains (including brown and wild rice and whole oats), pastas, flours, dried fruits, and nuts in the bulk sections of stores for far less. Organic brown rice in bulk is about 99 cents per pound.

When it comes to certain types of foods, here are the top organic picks on which to spend your dollars.

PRODUCE

The most important fruits and vegetables you should buy organic are those with the greatest pesticide residues and the ones you eat most often. Government lab tests show that even after washing, certain fruits and vegetables carry much higher levels of pesticides than do others.

Between 2000 and 2005, the not-for-profit Environmental Working Group (EWG) analyzed the results of nearly 51,000 tests for residues on produce. Based on the data, they created a "dirty dozen" list of the most contaminated fruits and veggies. Top offenders include: peaches, apples, bell peppers, celery, nectarines, strawberries, cherries, pears, grapes (imported), spinach, lettuce, and potatoes. Always buying these foods organic is ideal, but if you can't, focus on those you eat all the time.

Shop Smart

Buy organic produce in season (preferably local). Produce is at its most affordable when it's purchased in season. Sometimes you can save up to 50 percent.

Choose organic foods without fancy packaging. A bag of 10 2-ounce single-serving packets of organic baby carrots is $5, but for $3.50 less, you can buy a 1-pound bag of whole organic carrots. This veggie is not on the EWG's high-risk list, but if you buy carrots often, go organic.

MILK, YOGURT, AND CHEESE

Per half gallon, organic milk is more expensive—about $4 versus $2.50—but it's worth the splurge. Recent studies revealed impressive findings on organic milk. It contains 75 percent more beta-carotene—that's as much as in a serving of Brussels sprouts. It also has 50 percent more vitamin E, a powerful antioxidant that aids the immune system and fights cancer and heart disease. Plus it provides two to three times the antioxidants lutein and zeaxanthin, and about 70 percent more omega-3 fatty acids. And organic milk contains more conjugated linoleic acid (CLA). This good fat has been linked to numerous health benefits, including stronger immunity, less belly fat, a lower risk of type 2 diabetes, and healthier arteries.

Similar to meat, organic dairy contains no hormones or antibiotics, and there are no pesticides in the cows' feed. (In 2005, diphenylamine, a pesticide residue, was found in up to 92 percent of more than 700 conventional milk samples.) Current guidelines recommend three servings of dairy per day, and among organic choices, milk tends to be the most frugal option at about 50 cents per 1-cup serving (versus 31 cents for conventional). Organic cheese (about $1.30 per serving) and yogurt (about 60 cents per serving) are more costly.

Shop Smart

Download coupons. Many organic dairy companies such as Stonyfield Farm (stonyfield.com) and Organic Valley (organicvalley.coop) offer printable coupons on their sites for as much as $1 off a half gallon of milk or 16-ounce container of yogurt.

MEAT AND POULTRY

A study in the journal *Meat Science* compared the nutritional content of organic and nonorganic chicken meat. Researchers found the organic samples contained 28 percent more omega-3s, essential fatty acids that are linked to reduced rates of heart disease, depression, type 2 diabetes, high blood pressure, inflammation, and Alzheimer's disease. Animals raised organically can't be given antibiotics or growth hormones.

Shop Smart

Stretch it. The recommended portion size for meat and poultry is 3 ounces, the size of a deck of cards. Stick to this amount and round out your meal with less expensive whole grains and veggies to cut meal costs and improve nutritional balance. A pound of organic whole chicken for $4 with brown rice and in-season veggies can feed a family of four.

Become a "flexitarian." Choose beans as a protein source a few times a week. A 15-ounce can of organic beans is just $1.20, and a 1-cup serving provides 36 percent of your daily fiber needs. Bonus: Beans are some of the highest-ranking antioxidant foods.

Sign on. Watch videos about the best organic buys at Prevention.com/organicfood.

ON OUR RADAR

With the increased interest in organically grown food, there's a race among chemists to formulate safe pesticides made from natural materials, known as biopesticides.

One promising biopesticide contains an extract from the giant knotweed, a 12-foot weed that commonly grows along the East Coast. Compounds from the extract trigger the plants' own defenses to combat a range of diseases. The scientists say that the product is safe for humans, animals, and the environment. They plan to make the biopesticide available to organic commercial farmers this year.

HARNESS THE POWER OF "GOOD" BUGS

Probiotics strengthen immunity, ease digestion, and more. Here are the ones that will work well for you

It's official: After centuries of trying to sanitize and sterilize bacteria off the face of the planet, Americans have embraced the notion that some microbes might actually be good for us.

That's something Europeans have known for a long time. People in 35 countries around the world regularly down an immune booster called Actimel. Its French manufacturer, Danone, sells more than 1 billion single-serving bottles a year, or more than 2 million a day. And the Japanese have been tossing back a bacteria-laden drink called Yakult for more than 70 years.

Now Americans are running to the grocery store and supplement aisle to catch up. Dannon, the US subsidiary of Danone, sells Actimel here

THE BEST SUPPLEMENTS TO BUY

Probiotic products are multiplying nearly as fast as bacteria, but many contain bacteria that haven't performed well in studies, or haven't been tested. Others don't actually deliver the bugs they promise. A recent analysis by independent tester ConsumerLab.com found that out of 13 products tested, only 8 delivered at least 1 billion live organisms per serving (the generally accepted minimum).

The products below are reliable: They're recommended by probiotic researcher Gary Huffnagle, PhD, of the University of Michigan Medical School or Mary Ellen Sanders, PhD, executive director of the International Scientific Association for Probiotics and Prebiotics. Try one at a time to treat a problem. Although it's safe to double up, you won't know which product helps.

To Boost Your Immune System

BUY THIS BUG: *L. reuteri* SD2112 (also called *L. reuteri protectis* or Reuteri)

BY THIS NAME: Biogaia Probiotic chewable tablets

WHERE TO GET IT: biogaia.com

BUY THIS BUG: *L. rhamnosus GG* (also called Lactobacillus GG or LGG)

BY THIS NAME: Culturelle

WHERE TO GET IT: culturelle.com; (800) 722-3476

BUY THIS BUG: Blend of five bacterial strains

BY THIS NAME: Theralac

WHERE TO GET IT: theralac.com

under the name DanActive. And their Activia yogurt exploded onto the US market in 2006, racking up over $100 million in first-year sales.

Scientists have long known that bacteria play an important role in maintaining your health. Some 100 trillion microbes call the human body home. In your gastrointestinal tract, 500 to 1,000 different types of bac-

To Prevent Eczema and Allergies

BUY THIS BUG: *L. rhamnosus GG* (also called Lactobacillus GG or LGG)

BY THIS NAME: Culturelle

WHERE TO GET IT: culturelle.com; (800) 722-3476

To Relieve Irritable Bowel Syndrome

BUY THIS BUG: *B. infantis* (also called Bifantis)

BY THIS NAME: Align

WHERE TO GET IT: aligngi.com

BUY THIS BUG: *L. rhamnosus GG* (also called Lactobacillus GG or LGG)

BY THIS NAME: Culturelle

WHERE TO GET IT: culturelle.com; (800) 722-3476

BUY THIS BUG: *S. boulardii lyo*

BY THIS NAME: Florastor

WHERE TO GET IT: florastor.com

BUY THIS BUG: Blend of five bacterial strains

BY THIS NAME: Theralac

WHERE TO GET IT: theralac.com

To Ease Vaginal Infections

BUY THIS BUG: Blend of *L. reuteri RC-14* and *L. rhamnosus GR-1*

BY THIS NAME: Fem-Dophilus

WHERE TO GET IT: jarrow.com

teria help crowd out harmful germs, speed the digestion of food, and keep your immune system functioning properly.

But even though your body already hosts millions of "good" bugs, you could probably use a few more. In one study, researchers gave 94 employees of a Swedish company a daily dose of *Lactobacillus reuteri* (100 million "colony-forming units," or CFU) for 80 days. The workers used less than half as many sick days as did 87 employees who took a placebo. In other words, a probiotic a day kept the doctor away.

Probiotics will someday be recognized as "a new essential food group," predicts Gary Huffnagle, PhD, a professor of internal medicine at the University of Michigan Medical School and a prominent probiotics researcher. "I believe we'll eventually have research-based minimum daily requirements for probiotics," he says, "just as we do for many vitamins and minerals."

For now, it's clear that probiotics can help you get and stay healthy—if you take the right ones. Here's a guide to what they are, what they do, and how to get the biggest bang from your bugs.

PROBIOTICS' BENEFITS

You may be wondering, what can probiotics do for me? The simplest answer is: They can protect your stomach from a variety of ills. Research has shown that several types of bacteria are effective against diarrhea caused by viruses or antibiotics. And a British study found that women who took a daily dose of 100 million CFU of Bifidobacterium infantis (also called *B. infantis* or Bifantis) reduced symptoms of irritable bowel syndrome (IBS) by 20 percent more than those who took a placebo.

Gastroenterologist Charlene Prather, MD, MPH, an associate professor of internal medicine at Saint Louis University School of Medicine, now "prescribes" a probiotic capsule called Align to some of her patients with severe IBS. The condition had left some of them unable to travel or even attend kids' soccer games, but the probiotic "helps them do more of the things they want to do," Dr. Prather says.

Probiotics also seem to boost your immune system. A handful of studies show that they can shorten or prevent illness. Recent research points to a possible reason: A probiotic brew increased activity of natural killer cells—which are part of the immune system's early defense team against invaders.

That may be why two Lactobacillus strains (*L. reuteri* and *L. rhamnosus*) seem to help control vaginal infections. Last year, two reports showed that a supplement combining those strains, sold as Fem-Dophilus, helped get rid of bacterial vaginosis. Women taking medicine plus the supplement were twice as likely to be cured as women who took only the drug.

Studies suggest that other strains ease eczema and allergies. In Finland, researchers halved the incidence of eczema among babies by giving L. rhamnosus (also called Lactobacillus GG) to 77 mothers late in pregnancy, and then to the breastfeeding moms or to the infants for their first 6 months. Researchers suspect that the strain might help adults, too.

SHOP SMART

Not all bacteria survive the processing that dairy products undergo. The best way to ensure that refrigerated and frozen foods contain bacteria that withstand processing is to look for the National Yogurt Association's "Live & Active Culture" seal on the label. This seal indicates that refrigerated yogurt contained at least 100 million cultures and that frozen yogurt contained at least 10 million cultures per gram at the time they were manufactured.

"GUT BUGS" MAY REVOLUTIONIZE MEDICINE

Trillions of microbes live symbiotically in our guts, and we each have our own unique populations. Abnormal microbes have recently been linked to certain diseases, including diabetes and obesity. Scientists at the Imperial College of London found that they could alter gut bugs with probiotics. These results could lead to exciting possibilities in the prevention and treatment of diseases. The researchers believe it would be much safer and more efficient to treat diseases with drugs that change the flora of our digestive systems instead of treating the disease directly. These medications would be tailored to the patients' microbes, making the drugs more effective and less likely to cause side effects, say the scientists.

PROBIOTIC FOODS VS. PILLS

For overall health, eat your bacteria; you'll get a variety of bugs and benefits. Yogurt's your best bet: It always contains *S. thermophilus* and *L. bulgaricus*. Many brands also contain *L. acidophilus*. Some include still other strains; look for one that adds bifidobacterium to the three above, says Huffnagle, author of *The Probiotics Revolution*. If you eat a balanced diet, 6 to 8 ounces daily is plenty. Need help with a specific health condition, such as IBS? Take a supplement, too. (See "The Best Supplements to Buy" on page 118.)

If you decide to take probiotic pills instead, make sure you get the right bacteria for your needs. (See "The Best Supplements to Buy on page 118 for reliable strains.) Then check that the supplement contains a minimum of 1 billion CFU.

fast fact
160: The number of miles Mary Chervenak's relay team will run each day (See related story on next page.)

HEALTH HEROES

She's Bringing Hope— and Clean Water—to 1.1 Billion People

On June 1, Mary Chervenak, 39, embarked on the 2007 Blue Planet Run—the first-ever 20-member relay through 16 countries in 95 days. The goal: to raise awareness about unclean drinking water, which causes 80 percent of the world's illnesses.

"One in six people doesn't have safe water; women and children haul buckets 6 hours to their homes," says the Winston-Salem, North Carolina, chemist and 13-time marathoner, who collects donations along the route. "Just $35 can give someone access for life."

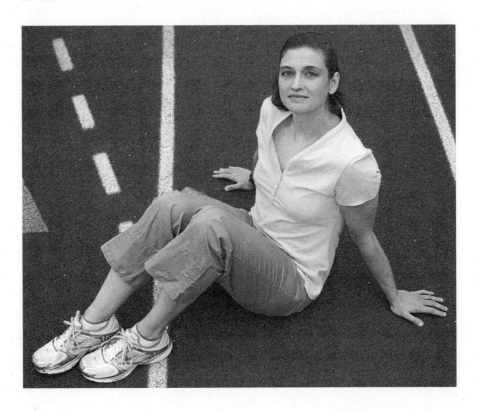

PART

III

WEIGHT-LOSS WISDOM

CHAPTER 15

WELCOME BACK CARBS

Why eating carbs can help you slim down—and how to do it right

Potatoes get a bad rap as little more than a waist-thickening waste of calories. But amazing new research puts spuds squarely at the center of the latest weight-loss buzz, along with other unfairly maligned carbs such as corn and rice. The reason: All of these foods contain resistant starch, which is a unique kind of fiber you'll be hearing a lot more about. In fact, experts agree that it's one of the most exciting nutrition breakthroughs they've seen in years.

"Resistant starch has the potential to become the next hot nutrition trend," says Leslie Bonci, RD, author of the *American Dietetic Association Guide to Better Digestion*. Indeed, more than 160 studies have examined this little-known nutrient's remarkable health and weight-loss benefits.

RESISTANT STARCH: THE NEW POWER NUTRIENT

Although this may be the first you've heard of resistant starch, it's likely been a part of your diet most of your life. Resistant starch is a type of dietary fiber naturally found in many carbohydrate-rich foods such as potatoes, grains, and beans, particularly when these foods are cooled (such as potato salad, cooked-and-cooled pasta, and cold rice in sushi). It gets its name because it "resists" digestion in the body, and though this is true of many types of fiber, what makes resistant starch so special is the powerful impact it has on weight-loss and overall health. As a dieter's tool it can't be beat: It increases your body's ability to burn fat, and it also fills you up and reduces overall hunger. Its health benefits are truly impres-

SIX BEST FAT-BURNING FOODS

TRY	RESISTANT STARCH	SMART SERVING SUGGESTIONS
Beans	8 grams per ½ cup	▪ Snack on chilled pinto bean dip with crudités. ▪ Substitute hummus for mayo on sandwiches. ▪ Add black beans to garden salads.
Bananas (slightly green)	6 grams per small	▪ Slice and mix with yogurt and oats for breakfast. ▪ Dip in yogurt, roll in chopped nuts, and freeze as an ice-cream alternative. ▪ Dice and toss with lemon juice, salt, sugar, and onion to make tangy banana chutney.
Potatoes and yams	4 grams per ½ cup	▪ Serve cold potato salad as a side dish. ▪ Add chilled, chunked red potatoes to a salad. ▪ Puree cooked white potatoes to create a chilled garlic potato soup.
Barley	3 grams per ½ cup	▪ Add to chilled lentil salad. ▪ Mix into tuna, chicken, or tofu salad. ▪ Sprinkle onto garden salads.
Brown rice	3 grams per ½ cup	▪ Order brown rice sushi. ▪ Mix chilled brown rice with fat-free milk, raisins, and cinnamon in place of cold cereal for breakfast. ▪ Add to chilled marinated cucumbers as a side dish.
Corn	2 grams per ½ cup	▪ Add to a taco salad, burrito, or quesadilla. ▪ Sprinkle into salsa. ▪ Make fresh corn relish.

sive as well. Studies show it improves blood sugar control, boosts immunity, and may even reduce cancer risk.

Resistant starch is bulky, so it takes up space in your digestive system. And because you can't digest or absorb it, the starch never enters your bloodstream. That means it bypasses the fate of most carbohydrates, which get socked away as body fat when you eat more than you can burn. Here are two more key ways resistant starch can help you drop unwanted pounds.

It ups your calorie burn. Unlike some types of fiber, resistant starch gets fermented when it reaches the large intestine. This process creates beneficial fatty acids, including one called butyrate, which may block the body's ability to burn carbohydrates.

"This can prevent the liver from using carbs as fuel and, instead, stored body fat and recently consumed fat are burned," explains Janine Higgins, PhD, nutrition research director for the University of Colorado Adult and Pediatric General Clinical Research Center. In your body, carbohydrates are the preferred source of fuel, similar to gasoline that powers your car's engine. Butyrate essentially prevents some of the gas from getting into the tank, and your cells turn to fat as an alternative. One study found that replacing just 5.4 percent of total carbohydrate intake with resistant starch created a 20 to 30 percent increase in fat burning after a meal.

It shuts down hunger hormones. Animal studies have found that resistant starch prompts the body to pump out more satiety-inducing hormones. A meal with resistant starch triggers a hormonal response to shut off hunger, so you eat less. Research shows that you don't reap this benefit from other sources of fiber.

FIGHTING DISEASE, ONE POTATO AT A TIME

The research on resistant starch doesn't stop at weight-loss. This powerful nutrient is also earning accolades as a major disease fighter from

(*continued on page 132*)

FIVE FOOD FIXES FOR FLAT ABS

You can't down 3,000 calories a day and expect to lose your belly, but calories aren't the entire story. Certain foods seem to pack pounds on the midsection: Experts from the ongoing Framingham Nutrition Studies reported that women who ate almost 400 fewer daily calories but chose the least nutritious foods had a 2½ times higher risk of abdominal obesity than those who ate that much more but made better choices. They also had a dramatically higher risk of such serious health issues as type 2 diabetes and heart attacks, says Barbara Millen, DPH, the study's director of nutritional research. You don't have to "diet"; just fold these strategies into your life and watch ab flab pare down.

EAT FRUITS AND VEGETABLES. Especially orange ones. Women trimmed their waists by replacing refined grains such as white bread and simple or added sugar with carbs from fruits and vegetables, according to a review from Copenhagen University Hospital in Denmark.

Besides packing in the fiber, which keeps you feeling full longer, researchers suspect it's the rich antioxidants, such as vitamin C and beta-carotene, that ward off ab fat. Carrots, cantaloupe, squash, and peaches are great sources of beta-carotene, while oranges, berries, and kiwifruit provide a good dose of C. To keep calories down, pick veggies, such as bell peppers, before fruits, and choose fruits over juices.

GET MORE SELENIUM. This cancer-fighting mineral is also linked to lower rates of abdominal obesity, according to a survey of more than 8,000 Americans. People with low blood levels of selenium and other antioxidants had bigger waistlines than those with higher levels.

Selenium is found in many foods, but it can be hard to know whether you're getting the recommended 55 micrograms a day because amounts vary based on the soil in which food is grown and the feed livestock consume. To meet your requirement, try a supplement or eat a varied diet. Also, opt for foods grown in different areas, such as grains from the Midwest, Vermont cheeses, and nuts from California.

ADD SOME PROTEIN. Eating more protein keeps you full and boosts energy, which leads to overall weight-loss and—for those over 40—reduced ab fat in particular, according to finds from Skidmore College and Copenhagen University Hospital.

Aim to get 25 percent of your calories from protein. If you eat 2,000 calories a day, that's 500 from protein. Just make lean choices such as low-fat yogurt, fat-free milk, fish, and poultry. Nuts are another great source, but they can be high in calories. Have just five 1-ounce servings a week. An ounce is about 24 almonds, 18 cashews, or 35 peanuts.

DRINK A GLASS OF WINE A DAY. Don't start drinking wine just to fight ab fat, but if you enjoy a glass with dinner, it's a great benefit. Some studies even suggest that light to moderate drinking protects against female midsection weight gain, compared with teetotaling. Based on a review of data collected by the National Center for Health Statistics, one 4-ounce glass of red or white wine most days a week (up to 20 a month) seems to be best.

More, however, is not better. That extra glass of wine—or even just one cocktail—adds inches, found the Copenhagen study, while other research implicates beer in the proverbial "beer belly."

EAT THE RIGHT FATS. Research from Spain shows it's easier to stay slim eating monounsaturated fats (such as olive oil) and omega-3s (found mostly in fish but also in flaxseed and walnut oils and tofu), while omega-6 fats (prevalent in cereals, corn oil, baked goods, and eggs) cause ab fat to pile on.

Fats that should be eliminated completely: trans fats, which have no nutritional value and are mostly found in calorie-dense baked goods and chips. In a Wake Forest University study, monkeys eating a typical American diet for 6 years gained the human equivalent of 10 pounds more when the fat they ate was all trans fat, compared with those eating monounsaturated fat. Worse, "30 percent more fat was added in the abdominal region, and they had early signs of diabetes," says researcher Kylie Kavanagh, DVM.

Only 5 percent of people on carbohydrate-restricted diets manage to
keep the weight off after 2 years. Nutrition experts say the success rate
is low because these diets don't address addictive eating impulses.
----

standard bearers such as the World Health Organization. Here's why scientists around the globe are so excited about its health benefits.

It may prevent cancer. Research shows that the butyrate created by resistant starch may protect the lining of the colon, making it less vulnerable to the DNA damage that triggers diseases, such as colon cancer. It can also create a pH drop inside the colon, which boosts the absorption of calcium and blocks the absorption of cancer-causing substances.

It may fight diabetes and heart disease. Similar to other fibers, resistant starch helps control blood sugar levels. "Because it skips routine digestion, we see lower blood sugar and insulin levels following a resistant starch–rich meal," says Christine Gerbstadt, MD, RD, CDE, spokesperson for the American Dietetic Association. Blood sugar control translates into more energy and sustained energy. It also means long-term heart protection, because chronic high levels of blood sugar and insulin cause delicate arteries to become clogged and harden.

It boosts your immune system. "When you have low levels of good-for-you bacteria in your digestive system, it's very difficult to fight off disease," says Joanne Slavin, PhD, RD, a nutrition professor at the University of Minnesota. Resistant starch may boost the growth of probiotics, the same kind of healthy bacteria found in yogurt that keep bad bacteria in check.

HOW TO EAT ENOUGH

Right now, there is no specific target for resistant starch intake. But preliminary data show that the average American woman consumes about 4 grams of resistant starch each day. Experts such as Dr. Gerbstadt believe the research is strong enough to advocate doubling that.

Adding just ½ to 1 cup of cooled resistant starch–rich food per day can

HEALTH HEROES

By Feeding the Homeless, Her Patients Start to Nourish Themselves

On a cold night in Naperville, Illinois, people struggling with eating disorders face their fear: handling food. But they knead dough and chop veggies because this meal isn't just for them—it's for homeless people, too.

"The impact is powerful," says Maria Rago, PhD, 42, clinical director of the eating disorders program at Linden Oaks Hospital. "They see how lucky they are." Once, a teen patient burst into tears, afraid to take a bite; a homeless man comforted her. "Everyone ate that night," she says.

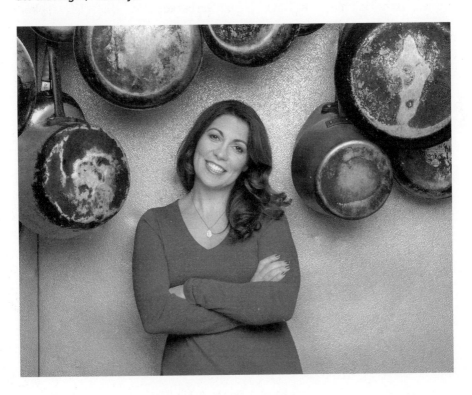

do the trick. See "Six Best Fat-Burning Foods" on page 128 for ideas, and follow this advice to maximize your intake.

Keep it cool. In cooked starchy foods, resistant starch is created during cooling. Cooking triggers starch to absorb water and swell, and as it slowly cools, portions of the starch become crystallized into the form that resists digestion. Cooling either at room temperature or in the refrigerator will raise resistant starch levels. Just don't reheat. That breaks up the crystals, causing resistant starch levels to plummet.

Look for fortified foods. A growing number of commercial foods have been bolstered with Hi-maize, which is the brand name of a resistant starch powder made from corn. You can use it in baking (and lower calories) by replacing up to one-quarter of traditional flour in any recipe without affecting taste or texture (King Arthur Hi-maize Natural Fiber, $5.95 per 12-ounce bag; kingarthurflour.com). Or look for packaged products that include Hi-maize as another easy way to boost your intake.

BREAK YOUR FAST

If you want to shed pounds and keep them off, then don't skip breakfast! Eating a breakfast with healthy proteins and a moderate amount of carbohydrates helps dieters lose weight and maintain their weight-loss.

Researchers at the Commonwealth University in Richmond, Virginia, compared the results of two low-calorie, low-fat diets. One diet allowed only 7 grams of carbohydrates and 12 grams of protein for breakfast, and the other diet allowed for 58 grams of carbs and 47 grams of protein.

After 4 months both groups of dieters lost about the same amount of weight. However, after 8 months, the low-carb dieters regained an average of 18 pounds while those on the "big breakfast" diet continued to lose weight. Furthermore, the women following the higher-carb diet felt fuller and had fewer cravings than the low-carb group did.

LOSE WEIGHT AFTER 40

Your three-step plan to trim
extra calories without counting,
dieting, or feeling deprived

Fat makes you fat. No, wait, carbs are the enemy. The truth is, when it comes to losing weight, it's all about calories: You have to burn off more than you take in to shed pounds. But over the years, that message has gotten lost, which may be partially to blame for our increased calorie consumption. Women now eat 22 percent more calories than they did in 1971, for an average of 1,877 per day. That may sound low, but only 19 percent of adults are highly active. This means that few women burn enough calories to warrant the amount they eat. (The lowdown: Every pound of body weight burns through 10 to 15 calories daily; only 10 if you're inactive, but up to 15 if you exercise 30 to 60 minutes most days.)

When you're guessing how many calories you can eat, being off by just 100 calories a day can keep you 6 to 10 pounds overweight. Experts say this is precisely why women in their forties are 25 pounds heavier now compared with 1960, and it's also why getting calories right is the only way to reach your ideal weight. Our guide will show you how.

STEP 1:
FIND OUT HOW MANY CALORIES YOU EAT

Women often underestimate how much they really eat, so follow these suggestions.

Track, don't count. You don't need to become a human calculator, but you should get a baseline idea of what you're consuming every day. A survey of more than 1,000 people found that only 13 percent knew how many calories they eat a day. The best way is to record each morsel you take in, for a day or two. Use our free journal at Prevention.com/health-trackers to jot down your diet.

Getting a grasp on exactly what you're eating can help you find out where the bulk of your calories comes from. Then you can make simple substitutions that shave off calories without sacrificing taste or satisfaction. For example, trading a handful of pretzels for 3 cups of air-popped popcorn sprinkled with 1 tablespoon of grated Parmesan cheese saves you about 115 calories and has loads more flavor while also tripling your portion size.

Read labels right. The Nutrition Facts info on a package lists the calorie count in one serving. But don't forget to compare that with the amount you actually eat or drink. Many packages contain two servings or more. For example, a 20-ounce bottle of organic lemonade contains 110 calories per serving, and 2½ servings per bottle. Drink the whole thing, and you racked up 275 calories. That's nearly 20 percent of a day's calorie needs for most women.

Look for total calories, not type. Surveys show that women look at grams of fat and sugar before calories, which is a habit that can mislead you into eating more than you should—especially when it comes to reduced-fat or low-sugar foods. For example, three regular Chips Ahoy! cookies provide 160 calories. Four of the reduced-fat version have 200. And sugar-free doesn't mean calorie-free. Five tiny Hershey's sugar-free dark chocolate candies provide 190 calories, and 1 cup of Edy's no-sugar-added Caramel Chocolate Swirl ice cream contains 220.

STEP 2:
DETERMINE HOW MANY CALORIES YOU NEED

Knowing your ideal goal prevents weight gain—and helps you lose. Use this simple equation to find your daily calorie needs.

Multiply your weight goal by 10 if you don't exercise at all, by 13 if you rarely exercise or only play the occasional weekend golf or tennis game, or by 15 if you regularly exercise (swim, walk, or jog) for 30 to 60 minutes most days of the week. The result is your total daily calories. Aim for this number every day to reach and maintain your weight goal.

For example, if your goal weight is 150 pounds, and if you rarely exercise, multiply 150 by 13 to get a total daily calorie allotment of 1,950.

To up your daily calorie allotment, move more. Going from being inactive to walking your dog every other day means you can multiply your weight goal by 13 rather than 10. For a 150-pound woman, that's an increase of 450 calories per day: So you could add one slice of whole wheat toast, 1 tablespoon of almond butter, 1 cup of grapes, and ¼ cup of semi-sweet chocolate chips to your daily diet without gaining.

fast fact ---

Forty percent of those who say they are trying to lose weight are not making an effort to reduce the calories they consume.

STEP 3: MAKE SMART CHOICES ALL DAY

It's easier than you think. Consider the following sample menu. The meals total 1,600 calories, the number most moderately active women need per day to support a healthy weight. Then check out the healthy tips that follow.

Breakfast: 8 ounces fat-free latte; 1 large tangerine; Egg Sandwich: 1 whole wheat English muffin, 1 egg scrambled in 1 teaspoon canola oil, 1 slice reduced-fat Cheddar cheese, ¼ avocado (sliced), 4 cherry tomatoes (halved). Total calories: 498

Lunch: 6 ounces fat-free strawberry yogurt; Garden Salad with Chickpeas: 1 cup salad greens, ¼ cup shredded red cabbage, 10 baby carrots, 5 yellow cherry tomatoes (halved), ½ cup chickpeas (or 3 ounces grilled skinless chicken breast), 2 tablespoons chopped walnuts, 2 tablespoons reduced-fat Italian dressing. Total calories: 479

Dinner: ½ cup steamed edamame; ¾ cup brown rice; Shrimp Stir-Fry: 15 large shrimp, 1½ cups broccoli stir-fried, 2 teaspoons peanut oil, 1 teaspoon low-sodium soy sauce, 1 teaspoon minced garlic, 1 teaspoon minced ginger. Total calories: 493

Snack: 1 cup green and red grapes. Total calories: 104

Healthy Tips

These tips were based on the preceding sample menu; apply them to your overall healthy diet.

Opt for whole fruit over juice. One cup of orange juice has more than 2½ times the calories of the tangerine. Plus, it's totally portion controlled.

Choose bread with holes in it. There's more air (and fewer calories!) in an English muffin, for example.

Have only one high-fat food per meal. High-fat foods (such as full-

WEEKEND WEAKNESS

Saturdays are hazardous to our waistlines. At least that's what the results of a study at Washington University School of Medicine suggest. Researchers analyzed the weight, activity, and food intake of 48 people for 1 year to see whether maintaining a low-calorie diet over a long period of time would slow down aging and disease.

The researchers divided the participants into three groups. The first group lowered their calorie intake by 20 percent. The second group increased their daily activity by 20 percent. And the last group didn't make any lifestyle changes.

The people who reduced their calories ate more on Saturdays. Those who increased their exercise ate more on Saturdays and Sundays. As a result, the group that dieted lost weight throughout the week and stopped losing weight on the weekends. The group that exercised actually gained weight on the weekends. The participants didn't always realize that they ate more on the weekends.

The researchers hoped that the results would mimic earlier findings that low-calorie diets extended the life span of rodents. "But rats don't have weekends like people do," they said.

fat dressing, nuts, croutons, or cheese) pack more calories into a smaller serving, which adds up quickly.

Make veggies half the bulk of your meals. Produce contains a lot of water, which makes it naturally low in calories.

Pick "slippery" salad dressings. Oil and vinegar or reduced-fat vinaigrette coat your salad more easily than thick ones such as blue cheese or Russian, so you can use less.

Always measure these foods: rice, cereal, peanut butter, and oil. They're hard to eyeball and are calorie dense. A heaping cup of rice has 25 percent more calories than a level one does.

Snack on a baseball-size portion of fresh fruit. It provides 50 to 100 calories, the amount in only three pretzel twists.

LISTEN UP
TO LOSE

Tuning in to your normal hunger
signals will ensure that you never
overeat again. Follow this six-step plan

Humans have an instinctual (even good) fear of getting hungry. Take the film *Into the Wild*. When the main character can't find food, his hunger drives him to a screaming, shake-his-fist-at-the-heavens rage, a stark example of the primal nature of our need for nourishment.

Today, most of us know where our next meal is coming from, yet our reaction to hunger has not evolved with our convenience-centered world. This is why even the *thought* of being hungry may send you running to the mini-mart for sustenance.

If you want to lose weight, however, you must tune in to your body's signal to eat. "Hunger is a physical clue that you need energy," says Dawn Jackson Blatner, RD. It can be your best diet ally. If you listen to your body, you'll instinctively feed it the right amount. But fall out of touch, and hunger becomes diet enemy number one: You may eat *more* than you need or get *too* hungry and stoke out-of-control cravings.

THE FRENCH PARADOX

When it comes to that second serving of pie, the French are quicker to say "uncle" than Americans are. For years scientists have been studying the "French Paradox:" How do the French stay so slim on a diet of rich sauces, cheese, bread, and pastries? Researchers at Cornell University believe it's because they listen to their internal cues, rather than the external cues to tell them when they are full. The French tend to stop eating when they feel full.

Many Americans are likely to rely on visual cues to signal fullness. For example Americans will stop eating when their beverage glass is empty, or their plate is clean, or when the TV show they're watching is over.

The following six tips will teach you how to spot hunger and eat to stay satisfied—so you control calories and shed pounds without "dieting."

LOCATE YOUR SPOT ON THE HUNGER SCALE

Do you really know what hunger feels like? Before you can rein it in, you must learn to recognize the physical cues that signal a true need for nourishment. Prior to eating, use the following hunger scale below to help figure out your true food needs.

Starving: This uncomfortable, empty feeling may be accompanied by light-headedness or jitteriness caused by low blood sugar levels from lack of food. Your risk of bingeing is high.

Hungry: Your next meal is on your mind. If you don't eat within the hour, you enter dangerous "starving" territory.

Moderately hungry: Your stomach may be growling, and you're planning how you'll put an end to that nagging feeling. This is optimal eating time.

Satisfied: You're satiated—not full, but not hungry either. You're relaxed and comfortable and can wait to nosh.

Full: If you're still eating, it's more out of momentum than actual hunger. Your belly feels slightly bloated, and the food does not taste as good as it did in the first few bites.

FIVE REASONS YOU OVEREAT—AND HOW TO STOP

YOU'RE HUNGRY BECAUSE	SOLUTION
There's no time in the morning for breakfast, so you grab a muffin or doughnut.	Zap a packet of instant oatmeal with low-fat milk as soon as you wake up. Take bites between showering, dressing, and grooming. Bring an apple or banana to eat in the car.
It's late afternoon, and you're low on energy. The office vending machine is calling your name.	Stash single-serving packages of nuts and dried fruit in your desk and plan to munch a few hours after lunch—when you feel moderate hunger.
You're going out for a late dinner with your friends, but it's only 5 p.m. and you're already hungry.	Have a 150- to 200-calorie snack such as yogurt with some fruit or celery and 2 tablespoons of peanut butter a couple of hours before your dinner date.
You've underestimated how long your errands would take; you're now ready for lunch but stuck in traffic.	Dig into your glove compartment for the high-fiber protein-packed bar you keep there for such emergencies. When you reach your destination, eat a lighter-than-normal lunch to compensate for the extra calories.
It's past your normal bedtime, and now your stomach is growling.	Grab a fiber-filled piece of low-calorie fruit such as a juicy apple or pear instead of, or at least before diving into, the cookie jar.

Stuffed: You feel uncomfortable and might even have mild heartburn from your stomach acids creeping back up your esophagus.

To slim down: The best time to eat is when you are "moderately hungry" or "hungry." When you hit either of these stages, you've used most of the energy from your last meal or snack, but you haven't yet hit the point where you will be driven to binge.

REFUEL EVERY 4 HOURS

Still can't tell what true hunger feels like? Set your watch. Moderate to full-fledged hunger (our ideal window for eating) is most likely to hit 4 to 5 hours after a balanced meal. Waiting too long to eat can send you on an emergency hunt for energy, and the willpower to make healthful choices plummets.

When researchers in the United Kingdom asked workers to choose a snack just after lunch, 70 percent picked foods such as candy bars and potato chips. The percentage shot up to 92 percent when workers chose snacks in the late afternoon. "Regular eating keeps blood sugar and energy stable, which prevents you from feeling an extreme need for fuel,"

THIS IS YOUR BRAIN ON HUNGER

Scientists are one step closer to understanding why certain people become obese and others do not. According to the *Journal of Neuroscience*, researchers in London developed a method using magnetic resonance imaging (MRI) to measure how full or hungry rodents feel. The researchers were able to see how neurons in the hypothalamus, where appetite is regulated, became very active when mice were hungry and then gradually slowed down as the mice ate.

This is exciting news in the study of obesity, which currently relies on subjective data to measure satiety, or that feeling of fullness. Scientists typically depend on participants to tell them how full they feel or study the food they eat in order to conduct research. This new method allows scientists to actually observe and define hunger in the brain, which will hopefully open up many more possibilities in the treatment of obesity.

says Kate Geagan, RD, a Park City, Utah–based register dietitian.

To slim down: If you're feeling hungry (see the scale on page 143) between meals, a snack of 150 calories should help hold you over. Here are a few ideas.

Munch on whole foods. For example, fruit and unsalted nuts tend to contain more fiber and water, so you fill up on fewer calories. Bonus: They're loaded with disease-fighting nutrients.

Pack snacks. Avoid temptation by packing healthful portable snacks such as string cheese and dried fruit in your purse, desk drawer, or glove compartment.

EAT BREAKFAST WITHOUT FAIL

A recent study published in the *British Journal of Nutrition* tracked the diets of nearly 900 adults. The researchers found that when people ate more fat, protein, and carbohydrates in the morning, they stayed satisfied and ate less over the course of the day than those who ate their bigger meals later on.

Unfortunately, many Americans start off on an empty stomach: In one recent survey, consumers reported that even when they eat in the morning, the meal is a full breakfast only about one-third of the time.

To slim down: If you're feeling full-blown hunger before noon, there's a chance you're not eating enough in the a.m. Aim for a minimum of 250 calories. Here's how to make it a habit.

Prepare breakfast before bed. Cut up some fruit and portion out some yogurt.

Stock your desk. Stash single-serving boxes of whole grain cereal or packets of instant oatmeal and shelf-stable fat-free milk or soy milk at work to eat when you arrive.

Eat a late breakfast if you can't stomach an early one. "Don't force anything," says John de Castro, PhD, a behavioral researcher and dean of the College of Humanities and Social Sciences at Sam Houston State University. "Just wait a while and eat at 9, 10, or even 11 a.m. It will help you stay in control later in the day."

BUILD LOW-CAL, HIGH-VOLUME MEALS

Solid foods that have a high fluid content can help you suppress hunger. "When we eat foods with a high water content like fruits and vegetables, versus low-water content foods like crackers and pretzels, we get bigger portions for less calories," says Barbara Rolls, PhD, author of *The Volumetrics Eating Plan* and a professor of nutritional sciences at Pennsylvania State University. Bottom line: You consume more food but cut calories at the same time. Rolls has found a similar effect in foods with a lot of air. In a recent study, people ate 21 percent fewer calories of an air-puffed cheese snack, compared with a denser one.

To slim down: Eat fewer calories by eating more food. Here are a few suggestions.

Start dinner with a salad. Or make it into your meal by adding some protein such as lean meat or beans.

Choose fresh fruit over dried. For around the same amount of calories, you can have a whole cup of fresh, succulent grapes or a measly 3 tablespoons of raisins.

Supplement frozen dinners. Boost the volume of a low-cal frozen dinner by adding extra veggies such as steamed broccoli or freshly chopped tomatoes and bagged spinach.

MUNCH FIBER ALL DAY LONG

Fiber can help you feel full faster and for longer. Because the body processes a fiber-rich meal more slowly, it may help you stay satisfied long after eating. Fiber-packed foods are also higher in volume, which means they can fill you up so you eat fewer calories. One review recently pub-

---

TRICK YOURSELF THIN

If you find it difficult to turn down that second plate of spaghetti, perhaps the plate is the problem! Studies have shown that the larger the plate, the bigger the serving of food, and the more likely we are to eat the entire serving. Simply putting your meals on a smaller plate can stop you from eating more than your body needs. Here are two more science-backed tips to help end mindless eating.

Use tall, thin glassware. Researchers discovered that when people use wide, short glasses, they drank up to 76 percent more than those who used tall, thin glasses.

When dining at a buffet, put your entire meal on one plate, including dessert. According to a Cornell University study, people who put all of the food they intended to eat on one plate ate 14 percent less than people who took smaller amounts and went back for two or three more servings.

---

lished in the *Journal of the American Dietetic Association* linked a high intake of cereal fiber with lower body mass index—and a reduced risk of type 2 diabetes and heart disease.

To slim down: Aim to get at least 25 grams of fiber a day.

Eat more produce. Fruits such as apples and vegetables such as carrots are naturally high in fiber. Eat some at each meal and snack.

Go whole grain. Try replacing some or all of your regular bread, pasta, and rice with whole-grain versions.

INCLUDE HEALTHY PROTEIN AT EACH MEAL

When researchers at Purdue University asked 46 dieting women to eat either 30 percent or 18 percent of their calories from protein, the high-protein eaters felt more satisfied and less hungry. Plus, over the course of 12 weeks, the women preserved more lean body mass, which includes calorie-burning muscle.

To slim down: Boost your protein intake with these ideas.

Go lean. Have a serving of lean protein such as egg whites, chunk light tuna, or skinless chicken at each meal. A serving of meat is about the size of a deck of cards or the palm of your hand.

Build beans into your meals. Black beans, chickpeas, and edamame (whole soybeans) are low in fat, high in fiber, and packed with protein.

OUTSMART YOUR CRAVINGS

What's behind your all-consuming desire for a cupcake? Science puts you back in control

One minute, you're innocently going about your day. The next, you're in the clutches of desire. Your object of lust: a chocolate cupcake with buttercream icing. Next thing you know, you're licking frosting off your fingers. What just happened?

You were clobbered by a craving. In a study from Tufts University, 91 percent of women said they experienced strong cravings. And willpower isn't the answer. These urges are fueled by feel-good brain chemicals such as dopamine, released when you eat these types of foods, which creates a rush of euphoria that your brain seeks over and over. What you need is a foolproof plan that stops this natural cycle—and, therefore, prevents unwanted weight gain.

The next time you're hit with an insatiable urge for a double-chocolate brownie, ask yourself the following four questions to get to the root cause, then follow our expert tips tailored to your trigger.

AM I STRESSED OUT?

When you're under pressure, your body releases the hormone cortisol, which signals your brain to seek out rewards. Comfort foods loaded with sugar and fat basically "apply the brakes" to the stress system by blunting this hormone, explains researcher Norman Pecoraro, PhD, who studies the physiology of stress at the University of California, San Francisco.

When you reach for food in response to negative feelings such as anger or sadness (for example, eating potato chips after a fight with your spouse), you inadvertently create a powerful connection in your brain. Remember Pavlov's dog? It's classic brain conditioning.

"The food gets coded in your memory center as a solution to an unpleasant experience or emotion," says Cynthia Bulik, PhD, author of *Runaway Eating* and director of the Eating Disorders Program at the University of North Carolina at Chapel Hill. Face that same problem again, and your brain will likely tell you, "Get the Cheetos!"

Do This!

Stimulate happiness. "Women especially have a profound emotional reaction to music," notes Bulik. She asks her clients to create upbeat playlists to listen to whenever a craving strikes. The songs provide a distraction and an emotional release.

Wait it out. "People give in to cravings because they think they'll build in intensity until they become overwhelming, but that's not true," says Bulik. Cravings behave like waves: They build, crest, and then disappear. If you can "surf the urge," you have a better chance of beating it altogether, she says.

Choose the best distraction. "What you're really craving is to feel better," says Linda Spangle, RN, a weight-loss coach in Broomfield, Colorado, and author of *100 Days of Weight-loss*. You've heard the trick about phoning a friend or exercising instead of eating. But taking a solo walk won't help if you're feeling lonely, says Laurie Mintz, PhD, a professor of counseling psychology at the University of Missouri. Instead, identify your current emotion—bored, anxious, mad—by filling in these blanks: "I feel ____ because of ____." Then find an activity that releases it. If you're stressed, channeling nervous energy into a workout can help; if you're upset over a problem at the office, call a friend and ask for advice.

HAVE I BEEN EATING LESS THAN USUAL?

If you're eating fewer than 1,000 calories a day or restricting an entire food group (such as carbs), you're putting your body in prime craving mode. Even just 3 days of strict dieting decreases levels of the appetite-reducing hormone leptin by 22 percent. Experts note that "restrained eaters"—dieters who severely limit calories or certain foods—aren't necessarily thinner than regular eaters. They're actually about 1 to 2 BMI points higher, or the equivalent of 10 to 20 pounds, because their self-imposed food rules often backfire.

According to research from the University of Toronto, restrained eaters are more likely to experience cravings and to overeat the "forbidden" food when given the chance. In a study published in the journal *Appetite*, women who were asked to cut their carbs for 3 days reported having stronger cravings and eating 44 percent more calories from carb-rich foods on day 4. "Making certain foods off-limits can lead to obsessing and bingeing," notes Kathy McManus, RD, director of nutrition at Brigham and Women's Hospital in Boston.

Do This!

Lift any bans—safely. Plan ways to enjoy your favorite foods in controlled portions, says McManus. Get a slice of pizza instead of a whole pie, or share a piece of restaurant cheesecake with two friends.

YOUR WORST DIET DAYS—SOLVED

You wouldn't watch Saturday morning cartoons on a Wednesday, and you wouldn't vote on a Friday. Well, there are certain days you probably won't be able to stick to a diet, either, found new research. Cornell University scientists say it's all in your mind-set.

"A Monday diet is usually a reaction to an indulgent weekend and can be too extreme and too limiting," says lead researcher Brian Wansink, PhD. The following science-proven tips will make your diet survive the days you're most tempted to give up.

MONDAY: Chips and dip, french fries, and cake, oh my. Your weekend was filled with junk food, and now you're in withdrawal. Eat veggies and fruits so you're not tempted to fill up on nutrient-poor snacks.

TUESDAY: Motivation flags: You dread making healthy changes all week and all year. Bribe yourself with scheduled snack times. Eat low-fat yogurt or a handful of almonds 1½ hours before a meal. Protein can take the edge off hunger.

FRIDAY: Weekend fun begins, and you can't refuse a dinner out with friends. Split a dish. Many are 1,000 calories or more; half is the perfect portion.

Don't "eat around" cravings. Trying to quell a craving with a low-cal imitation won't satisfy your brain's memory center, says Marcia Levin Pelchat, PhD, a researcher at Monell Chemical Senses Center in Philadelphia. For example, if you're craving a milkshake, yogurt won't cut it—especially if you've been depriving yourself. You may even take in more calories than if you'd just had a reasonable portion of what you wanted in the first place. Munching five crackers, a handful of popcorn, and a bag of pretzels, all in the name of trying to squash a craving for potato chips, will net you about 250 more calories than if you'd eaten a single-serving bag of chips.

AM I GETTING ENOUGH SLEEP?

In a University of Chicago study, a few sleepless nights were enough to drop levels of the hormone leptin (which signals satiety) by 18 percent and boost levels of ghrelin, an appetite trigger, by about 30 percent. Those two changes alone caused the participants' appetites to kick into overdrive and their cravings for starchy foods such as cookies, potato chips, and bread to jump 45 percent.

Do This!

Have some caffeine. It can help you get through the day without any high-calorie pick-me-ups. It won't solve your bigger issue of chronic sleep loss, but it's a good short-term fix until you get back on track.

Portion out a serving. You probably don't have the energy to fight it, so try this trick: Before you dig in, dole out a small amount of the food you want (on a plate) and put the rest away.

AM I A CREATURE OF HABIT?

You may not realize it, but seemingly innocent routines, such as eating cheese popcorn while watching TV, create powerful associations. "The brain loves routine," says Robert Maurer, PhD, author of *One Small Step Can Change Your Life*. The thought of letting go of these patterns can cause a fear response in an area of the brain known as the amygdala.

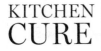

KITCHEN CURE

Your favorite fragrance can help manage your cravings. In a study at the Smell and Taste Research Foundation in Chicago, people who sniffed banana, green apple, and peppermint when they felt a craving lost more weight than non-sniffers did. So keep a bottle of your favorite scent handy throughout the day and sniff when cravings hit.

"Once the food hits your lips, the fear response shuts off in a heartbeat," says Maurer.

Do This!

Eliminate sensory cues. Smells, sights, and sounds all act as powerful triggers. Watch television in your basement or bedroom so you're far away from the kitchen and the cupboard full of snacks.

Picture yourself healthy. Try Maurer's "stop technique": Every time the food you crave pops into your head, think, Stop! Then, picture a healthy image (say, you lean and fit). After a while, your brain will dismiss the food image and the craving will subside. "One of my clients did this four or five times a day, and within 2 weeks, she stopped turning to sweets every night after dinner," he says.

Shift your focus. Australian researchers found that distracting your brain really does work. When a craving hits, divert your attention to something visual not related to food, such as typing an e-mail.

LOSE THE LAST 10 POUNDS

A few simple adjustments are all it takes to finally meet your weight-loss goal

You've cleaned up your diet, sweated off countless calories, and watched pounds melt away. But now the scale has come to a screeching halt. What gives? It's an unfortunate law of weight-loss: The last 10 pounds are harder to shed than the first 30.

That's because the slimmer you become, the fewer calories you burn just going about your day, explains Madelyn Fernstrom, PhD, founding director of the Weight Management Center at the University of Pittsburgh Medical Center and author of *Runner's World Runner's Diet*. For every pound you lose, your metabolism slows by up to 20 calories a day.

But we do have some good news: Easy tweaks to the good habits you've already established can push you past your plateau and help you reach your final weight-loss goal.

HEALTHY HABIT: DOING CARDIO FOUR OR FIVE TIMES A WEEK

Speed results: Do interval training three times a week.

Cardio melts calories, but to keep seeing results, ramp up your intensity, too. Canadian researchers found that when women did 10 sets alternating a 4-minute burst of intense cycling followed by 2 minutes of easy pedaling, they burned up to 66 percent more fat during subsequent aerobic workouts.

"Interval training can trigger a boost in metabolism so you burn more fat during low- and moderate-intensity activity, and even at rest," says Jason Talanian, PhD, a researcher at the University of Guelph in Ontario and coauthor of the study.

You can apply this principle to any workout, whether you're power walking, jogging, or using an elliptical machine: Alternate between a moderate effort that makes you slightly breathless and a vigorous pace that makes speaking more than a couple of words difficult. In a 30-minute interval workout, you'll burn 20 percent more calories than if you maintained a steady pace, and you'll keep burning more fat afterward. (For a fat-burning walking program, see chapter 21.)

HEALTHY HABIT: WALKING AS OFTEN AS POSSIBLE

Speed results: Stand an extra hour a day.

It's one of the dirtiest tricks your body can play: The more you exercise, the less you're inclined to stand, walk around, twiddle your thumbs, and generally burn calories during the 23 hours you're not working out. And small changes such as standing versus sitting can add up.

A study from Iowa State University found that obese women stood for 2 hours less than their lean counterparts, which is a simple habit that researchers say could make a difference of 300 calories a day.

Being aware of this potential pitfall can help you outsmart it, though. Standing for an hour more a day—at your desk, in the doctor's waiting room, or at your kids' soccer game—will burn 100 more calories than if you were sitting, says Darcy Johannsen, PhD, RD, a postdoctoral research associate. On the weekends, let your postworkout treat be window-shopping rather than movie watching to prevent a slump in calorie burn.

HEALTHY HABIT: WEARING A PEDOMETER

Speed results: Set a step goal.

Numerous studies show that wearing a pedometer can prompt you to be more active. To maximize your results, set goals and then track your progress. People given a specific step goal increased their walking distance by about a mile a day, while those without a target didn't alter their habits, finds a review of 26 studies in the *Journal of the American Medical Association*. Start by shooting for an extra 2,000 steps a day, working up to 10,000.

THE OBESITY DEMENTIA CONNECTION

Maintaining a normal body weight may stave off dementia, according to doctors at Johns Hopkins Bloomberg School of Public Health. An average person's risk of dementia is 1 in 10, but obesity raises that risk by 42 percent. Those extra pounds are linked to hypertension and may cause heart disease, which can damage blood vessels that lead to the brain.

That doesn't mean that being extra-slim reduces the chance of dementia. People who are underweight are at a 36 percent greater risk. Poor nutrition habits have been shown to impair memory and increase inflammation.

HEALTHY HABIT: LIFTING WEIGHTS

Speed results: Switch to circuit training.

Get a more time-efficient workout and burn a third more calories by doing strength and cardio in one shot. Cardio blasts calories immediately, while strength training increases metabolism over time, so combining the two gives you the ultimate bang for your buck, says *Prevention* advisory board member Wayne Westcott, PhD.

In a study led by Westcott, exercisers who did a 25-minute circuit routine (alternating 1 minute of weights with 1 minute of cycling) three times a week for 12 weeks trimmed their waistlines by 4 percent. At home, do 1 minute of jumping jacks or easy rope jumping between every strength exercise.

HEALTHY HABIT: CUTTING OUT UNHEALTHY FATS

Speed results: Be a part-time vegetarian.

Eating less meat is a proven way to lighten up on the scale. Research shows that vegetarians weigh an average 20 percent less than nonvegetarians. George Washington School of Medicine researchers found that women who followed a vegan diet for 14 weeks lost two and a half times as much weight as those who limited fat intake.

You don't have to go cold turkey. Just eating less meat can make a difference. In a Brigham Young University study of 284 women, 53 percent of those who typically averaged about 10 ounces of meat a day were overweight, compared with 16 percent of those who ate less than 6 ounces.

Plant-based foods are naturally low in calories and high in nutrients and satiating fiber, so you feel full without overdoing it, says Gabrielle M. Turner-McGrievy, RD. A cup of lentil soup, a small handful of nuts, or ¼ cup of chickpeas tossed with whole wheat pasta and veggies are all good protein-rich swaps.

Not ready to nix meat altogether? Start by trying three vegetarian dinners a week for a month to allow your taste buds to adjust. And trust us, they will. In another weight-loss study of new vegetarians versus low-fat dieters, a third more of the vegetarians had stuck with the diet a year later.

HEALTHY HABIT: BOXING UP HALF YOUR ENTRÉE

Speed results: Munch a pre-meal apple.

An apple a day could keep the pounds away, suggest Pennsylvania State University researchers. Diners who had an apple 15 minutes before an all-you-can-eat pasta lunch ate 187 fewer calories than those who skipped the snack. At 65 calories per cup, the apple fills you up.

"Starting a meal with a lower-calorie food leaves less room for

(continued on page 162)

KITCHEN CURE

Want to fire up your metabolism? Spice up your meals with chile peppers.

Capsaicin, the bioactive compound that makes chile peppers exude heat, can turn your metabolism up a notch while also enhancing satiety and reducing hunger. Studies show that eating about 1 tablespoon of chopped red or green chile pepper—which is equal to 30 milligrams of capsaicin—resulted in up to a 23 percent temporary boost in metabolism.

In another study, 9 milligrams of red pepper was given in capsule form or naturally in tomato juice before each meal. The researchers noted that the individuals reduced their total calorie intake by 10 or 16 percent, respectively, for 2 days after and still reported being full.

To wake up your metabolism—and your taste buds—sprinkle red pepper flakes onto pasta dishes and into chilis and stews. Fresh chile peppers work well in salsa and add a fiery flavor to many other dishes.

METABOLISM MYTHS—BUSTED

Google the word *metabolism*, and you'll find nearly 45 million results. The number of products that claim to boost your body's fat-burning capacity seems limitless.

There are probably more myths about metabolism than there are about the Loch Ness Monster and Bigfoot combined. The reality: Your body does burn 2 to 5 percent fewer calories with each decade after age 40, and women tend to put on about a pound a year as a result, but these changes are not inevitable, says Matt Hickey, PhD, director of the Human Performance Clinical Research Lab at Colorado State University. Making simple changes to your routine, such as those outlined in chapter 23, can up your calorie burn and compensate for the deficit, keeping you from succumbing to age-related weight gain. Here are the facts behind the metabolism folklore.

Drinking Water Can Help You Burn Calories

TRUE: All of your body's chemical reactions, including your metabolism, depend on water. If you are dehydrated, you may be burning up to 2 percent fewer calories, according to researchers at the University of Utah who monitored the metabolic rates of 10 adults as they drank varying amounts of water per day. In the study, those who drank either eight or twelve 8-ounce glasses of water a day had higher metabolic rates than those who drank four.

TIP: If your urine is darker than light straw in color, you may not be drinking enough fluid. Try sipping one glass before each snack and meal to stay hydrated.

Eating Protein Will Rev Up Your Metabolism

TRUE: Protein provides a metabolic advantage compared with fat or carbohydrates because your body uses more energy to process it. This is known as the thermic effect of food (TEF). Studies show that you may burn up to twice as many calories digesting protein as carbohydrates. In a typical diet, 14 percent of calories come from protein. Double that (and reduce carbs to make up for the extra calories), and you can burn an additional 150 to 200 calories a day, explains Donald Layman,

PhD, a professor of nutrition at the University of Illinois.

TIP: To reap protein's rewards, strive for between 10 and 20 grams at each of your meals, says Hickey. Try an 8-ounce cup of low-fat plain yogurt with breakfast (about 13 grams), a ½-cup serving of hummus with lunch (about 10 grams), and a 3-ounce salmon fillet for dinner (about 17 grams).

Lifting Weights Boosts Metabolism More Than Cardio

TRUE: When you strength-train enough to add 3 pounds of muscle, you increase your calorie burn by 6 to 8 percent—meaning that you burn about 100 extra calories every day. Aerobic exercise, on the other hand, doesn't significantly increase your body's lean muscle mass. "The best way to gain muscle mass is to do resistance training," notes Ryan D. Andrews, RD, a certified strength-training specialist in Colorado.

TIP: "You want to focus on exercises that recruit the largest muscles and use two-part movements, because they will help you build more lean mass," Andrews says. His favorites include squats, pushups, and any exercise that combines upper- and lower-body movements. For a metabolism-boosting strength-training workout, see chapter 23.

Celery Uses Up More Calories Than It Provides

FALSE: The thermic effect of food does cause your body to burn up calories as it processes meals, snacks, and beverages. But this process accounts for anywhere from 0 to 30 percent of the calories you eat. Protein, for example, takes more calories to digest than fat or carbohydrates. A medium-size rib of celery has only about 6 calories; its TEF is approximately half a calorie. In reality, "negative calorie foods" are nothing more than wishful thinking.

TIP: Include celery as a low-calorie but filling addition to salads, stir-fries, and soups. You can't depend on it to magically melt away your trouble spots, but it is healthful. Celery has phthalides, compounds that can help reduce blood pressure.

(continued)

high-calorie entrées, so you naturally eat less," says Julie Flood, PhD, a nutrition researcher formerly with Pennsylvania State University. Try a veggie platter with hummus or a tossed salad for a similar effect.

HEALTHY HABIT: WATCHING PORTION SIZE

Speed results: Be extra vigilant on weekends.

Shrinking portions is a no-brainer for weight-loss, but when it comes to zapping stubborn pounds, lax weekend habits could cause the scale to stick. Even dieters on calorie-controlled plans average an extra 420 calories a weekend (starting Friday night), finds a Washington University School of Medicine study—enough to stall weight-loss.

from being "hormonal" can equal as much as 300 calories a day, which is why their appetite increases during this phase.

TIP: Keep a journal of what you eat the week before and the weeks after your period. Try to maintain your eating pattern over the course of the month so that you can take advantage of this hormone-driven calorie burn. If you give in to cravings, make sure that you keep portions in check.

Exercise at a Higher Intensity for a Metabolic Afterburn

TRUE: People who exercise at very high intensities experience a postexercise boost in resting metabolic rate that is larger and lasts longer compared with those who work out at a low or moderate level. Up the effort of your workout and you can expect to burn at least 10 percent of the total calories used during the workout in the hour or so after exercising. So, if you do a combo of walking and jogging for 4 miles (about 400 calories) instead of just walking, you may burn an extra 40 calories in the next few hours.

TIP: Infuse your workout with bursts of speed. Gradually work your way up to 2-minute intervals, 3 days a week.

To be a weekend calorie warrior, avoid temptation at home and out. Using smaller plates could instantly cue you to eat less, research shows. Away from home, carry a healthy, portable snack (such as raw veggies) and steer clear of the food court.

HEALTHY HABIT: KEEPING A FOOD DIARY

Speed results: Track calories online.

Dieters who jotted down what they ate lost twice as much weight as those who didn't keep a record, research shows. Stay accountable by logging your meals and workouts for free at Prevention.com/healthtrackers. You'll also get colorful side-by-side graphs of your calorie balance.

PART

IV

FITNESS
TRAILBLAZING

START YOUR FITNESS PLAN ON THE RIGHT FOOT

Stick-with-it strategies to shed pounds and get strong—guaranteed

Want to boost your mood, fight off disease, manage your weight, sleep better, and put the spark back in your sex life? The answer's not in a pill; it's in your sneakers. If you're ready to start an exercise program, just making the commitment is an amazing first step. To ensure success, here are seven surprisingly simple, research-backed strategies that can help you overcome the most common roadblocks to weight-loss. They'll motivate you through the ups and downs of any new workout routine, so you'll stick to it and reach all your fitness goals.

BE COOL

Studies show that cooling your body temperature before you exercise can increase your stamina by 16 percent and even help you go faster. So hop in a swimming pool, take a cold shower, or soak your T-shirt in ice water to chill out *before* you work out.

LEARN WHAT "BUILD SLOWLY" MEANS

Be realistic about your abilities. The experts say to progress gradually, however most of us don't know how to translate that into real-life terms, especially those who used to be active but now have gotten out of the habit. "Formerly fit people are surprised and frustrated when they find themselves winded after a walk around the park," says Madelyn Fernstrom, PhD, founding director of the Weight Management Center at the University of Pittsburgh Medical Center.

If you haven't worked out in years, you must start with a manageable goal, such as 20 minutes of walking or yoga twice a week for 2 weeks. Then when you're ready to progress, either bump up your number of workouts to three a week or increase their length to 25 or 30 minutes, but don't try both at the same time. Taking on too much too soon can leave you achy and discouraged. That's why the experts strongly recommend you change only one thing at a time—the frequency, duration, or intensity of your workouts.

If your new cardio workout still leaves you gasping for air, don't be afraid to slow down your pace. Ideally, you should be slightly breathless but still able to talk without any trouble. Remember, you'll be more likely to follow your program if you exercise at a comfortable level. Strength training will get easier, too. In a new study from Ohio University, it was found that muscles adapt to resistance exercises after only a mere 2 weeks.

KEEP AN ACTIVITY LOG

Hands down, lack of time is the number one reason we struggle to keep exercising. Yet studies find that we may have more time than we think. Women ages 45 to 70 spend an average of 28 hours a week in sedentary activities outside of their jobs, such as reading and Web surfing, according to a University of Oklahoma study—ample time to find at least 2½ hours a week for exercise. First, keep a log of everything you do for 3 days, suggests Jennifer White, PhD, an assistant professor of fitness and

SHAKE THINGS UP

If your exercises have become "comfortable," then you may be in an exercise rut. It's time to step things up to keep you motivated and your muscles challenged! Here are three clues that your workout has the blues, and quick fixes to help you resuscitate your routine.

YOU DON'T SWEAT. Perform the same routine week after week, and your body will adapt, causing you to burn fewer calories. To challenge your muscles, choose a weight that needs your last ounce of strength to lift the final rep. Speeding up or lengthening your cardio workout will get your body in a fat-burning zone. You'll know you're there when you can't say the Pledge of Allegiance (31 words) without taking a deep breath.

YOU CAN DO YOUR ROUTINE BLINDFOLDED. Learning something new helps keep your mind engaged and gives different muscles a workout. If you're afraid you'll look silly in a dance class, try a DVD at home. Or freshen up a stale workout with a new iPod playlist full of upbeat, motivating tunes.

YOU FIND YOURSELF SLACKING OFF. Resolve to make your workouts just as important as a meeting, and schedule it. Studies show that morning exercisers are more likely to stick with a regimen. If getting up at 6 a.m. isn't in your genes, ease into an exercise routine: Lift hand weights while you watch the news, stretch before you shower, or take the dog for a walk around the block. Getting those feel-good endorphins flowing sets the tone for the rest of the day.

wellness at the University of Nebraska at Omaha. Then find creative ways to sneak activity into your day. The time you spend in front of the TV can now double as a stretching session; a cell phone headset allows you to power walk while you're on hold with the credit card company or customer service rep at the phone company.

PREPARE FOR POSTWORKOUT HUNGER

Exercise can boost metabolism for a few hours, but burning more calories can increase your appetite. To avoid the munchies after exercising (and eating back the calories you just burned), try to schedule workouts so that you have a meal within an hour afterward. Or save part of an earlier meal to eat during that time, says Fernstrom. Snacks combining carbohydrates and protein—such as a fig bar and fat-free milk, or cantaloupe and yogurt—are best to refuel muscles and keep you from feeling ravenous later on. If you still feel hungry, wait 10 to 15 minutes before eating more to make sure you're physically, not just mentally, hungry. Distract yourself while you wait: Keep your hands occupied by cleaning out a drawer or reading.

BE ALERT TO PRIME DROP-OUT TIME

About half of new exercisers quit in the first few months, research has found. But support, either one-on-one or in a group, can keep your momentum going. "Getting help specific to your particular issues is key," says Fernstrom. If you struggle with exercise, try finding (or even forming) a walking group at work or at your local Y. If you're goal-focused, signing up for an event, such as walking a half or full marathon, can be the carrot you need to stay on track.

TAKE BREAKS

Missed a workout? Don't worry: Your waistline won't notice. Brown University scientists found that people on a 14-week weight-loss program who took occasional breaks from working out lost an average of 7 pounds—

MEET LARGE WEIGHT-LOSS GOALS SAFELY

Losing more than 100 pounds can seem like a Herculean task, but following a safe routine that keeps you motivated will help you meet that task head on. Chris Freytag, *Prevention*'s fitness expert and author of *Prevention's Shortcuts to Big Weight-loss*, recommends taking these beginners' steps to build strength safely, zap calories, and boost health. (Make sure you get your doctor's okay before starting any exercise routine.)

SLOW AND STEADY. Surprise: Panting and wheezing *reduces* your odds of success. An Iowa State University study found that overweight people enjoyed walking more at a pace they chose than when researchers bumped up the intensity even 10 percent over that speed. Pick a level that feels good, and you'll be more likely to exercise regularly.

KEEP IT LOW IMPACT. Less stress on joints helps you avoid injuries, especially if you have a lot of weight to lose. Try walking. It's easy, affordable, and great for your heart *and* your waistline. Swimming, cycling, and elliptical training are also good joint-friendly options.

INCH UP GRADUALLY. Start slow with 10 minutes for 3 or 4 days a week, then increase your time by 5 minutes each week until you're clocking at least 30 minutes per session.

LISTEN TO YOUR BODY. Fatigue, burning in your muscles, and slight breathlessness are normal. But gasping for air, dizziness, fainting, nausea, and sharp or shooting pain are signals to stop exercising and check with your doctor.

about the same amount as those who never missed a day. "Just pick up again as soon as you can," says Fernstrom. In the long run, it's the habit, not the individual days, that matters. For help, sign up for a weekly e-mail health newsletter: People who did exercised 14 percent more and ate better than those who didn't get inbox reminders, reports a University of Alberta study. (To join our free *Best of Prevention* newsletter, which covers health, weight-loss, and fitness three times a week, visit the Web site Prevention.com/newsletters.)

SPLURGE—THEN GET UP AND MOVE

One date with a pint (or even two) of ice cream won't doom your weight-loss unless you let guilt keep you off track. In fact, French researchers discovered that obese exercisers who bicycled for 45 minutes 3 hours after a high-fat meal metabolized more stored belly fat than those who cycled on an empty stomach. Although bingeing on cookies before your next workout obviously won't help you slim down, the study is a good reminder that not all is lost when you stray from your diet. In fact, your body may even kick it up a gear to help with damage control. Instead of giving up when a celebratory dinner with friends sends your calorie count through the roof, suggest a postmeal stroll or dancing. The party moves away from the table, and the evening can continue with a fun activity that helps you move toward your weight-loss goal.

PUT THE TREADMILL IN AN ATTRACTIVE ROOM

If a workout bores you, don't do it. "Research shows that if you enjoy an exercise, you'll stay with it, so keep trying activities until you find something you like," suggests White. Or jazz up a ho-hum workout with music or audiobooks. Just don't try to exercise in some dark, dreary corner of the house. So many people make the mistake of consigning the treadmill to the basement, White says. You'll be more likely to use exercise equipment if it's in a pleasant space with good light and in easy reach of the radio and TV, such as the family room. It's worth investing in a home exercise space that's both functional and attractive, whether by spending a little extra on a treadmill you won't mind showing off or buying pretty baskets to store your workout DVDs and dumbbells.

fast fact

4: The number of the world's highest peaks that Wendy Booker has climbed. (See related story on next page.)

HEALTH HEROES

She aims to be the first person with MS to climb the Seven Summits

When Wendy Booker, a mother of three, was diagnosed with multiple sclerosis, her youngest asked, "Mommy, are you going to die?" That was all the motivation Booker, now 53, needed. Although doctors discouraged it, she began climbing, easing symptoms such as numbness with daily medication. The Massachusetts native challenges stereotypes about people with MS. She recently ascended Argentina's Mt. Aconcagua. All told, Booker has climbed four of the world's highest peaks. Next on her "big seven" list: Mt. Everest. "I want others with a chronic illness to go find their own mountains," she says.

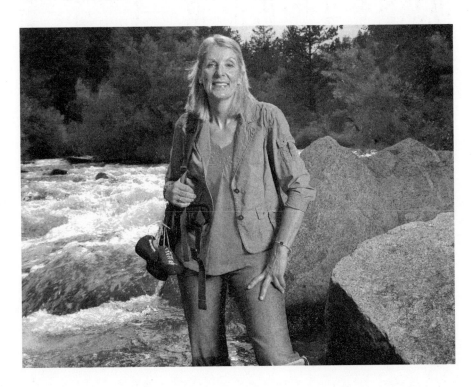

WALK OFF FIVE TIMES MORE WEIGHT

Blast calories plus trim and tone your trouble zones, with our fastest-ever routine

When it comes to walking, we know what you like: a simple, effective routine that fits into your life. Well, get ready for two plans you're gonna love: a 6-week fat-blasting plan and a walk-a-marathon (or half) program. These two workouts perfectly complement each other. Start with the 6-week program to get your body in tip-top walking shape. Then celebrate your success by signing up for a Team *Prevention* event at Prevention. com/team (it's a fun weekend away with *Prevention* editors and other readers) and begin following the marathon training plan. You'll be amazed at what your body can do!

Here's the really good news: Exercise scientists have discovered that shorter workouts can rev your metabolism higher and burn more fat than longer ones. The secret is intervals. In a study from the University of New South Wales in Australia, people who exercised 3 days a week for 20 minutes, alternating between fast- and moderate-paced intervals, lost five times as much weight—up to 20 pounds in 15 weeks without changing their diet—as those who exercised 3 days a week for 40 minutes at a steady, brisk speed. Even better, the interval exercisers shed most of the fat from their legs and belly.

Get ready to harness the fat-busting power of walking in two workouts!

OUR 6-WEEK FAT-BLASTING PLAN

This plan provides ultrafast results thanks to its three parts: (1) A variety of interval routines to challenge your muscles differently every day and keep your workouts fresh. "The race walkers I work with—who do lots of interval training—are slimmer now than when they were running," says Leigh Crews, certified trainer and spokesperson for the American Council on Exercise. (2) Endurance walks to make sure your overall calorie burn is high all week long. (3) Prewalk power moves to increase fat burn, build muscle, and speed your walking pace and metabolism. Start now and you can drop a dress size in just 6 weeks—without dieting!

Workout at a Glance

What you need: Supportive athletic shoes, 6-foot exercise band (available at sporting goods stores or online), watch with timer.

When to do it: 6 days a week. On three days, do the following intervals one per day to challenge your muscles and train your body to burn more calories. (The intervals are described in detail in the "6-Week Fat-Blasting Workout.")

Four by Twos will boost your endurance, so longer walks are a breeze.

30-Second Surges will increase your overall walking speed.

Even Stevens will improve your ability to go longer at top speeds.

On the other 3 days, you'll do Endurance Walks combined with our Prewalk Power Moves, which is a strength routine that builds muscle, boosts metabolism, and revs up the fat-burning power of these walks. (These moves are described in detail in "Prewalk Power Moves" on page 178.)

How to do it Follow these speed and intensity guidelines, based on a 1-to-10 scale (1 is sitting still, 10 is sprinting) for the workouts.

Easy pace (2.5 to 3 mph): 3 to 4 intensity level

Moderate pace (3 to 3.5 mph): 5 to 6 intensity level

Power pace (3.5 to 4 mph): 7 intensity level

Race pace (4 to 4.5 mph): 8 intensity level

Sprint (4.5 to 5 mph): 9 to 10 intensity level

6-Week Fat-Blasting Workout

Warm up by walking at an easy pace (level 3 to 4) for the first 4 minutes of each workout and do the same to cool down at the end (both are included in the total workout times listed in parentheses in the workout chart).

Endurance: Steady, moderate pace (level 5 to 6).

Four by Twos: Alternate 4 minutes of power pace walking (level 7) with 2 minutes of moderate pace walking (level 5 to 6).

30-Second Surges: Alternate 30-second sprints (level 9 to 10) with 1 minute of easy pace walking (level 3 to 4).

Even Stevens: Alternate equal amounts (see chart below for specifics) of race pace walking (level 8) with moderate pace walking (level 5 to 6).

	DAY 1	DAY 2	DAY 3	DAY 4	DAY 5	DAY 6
	Endurance	Four by Twos	Endurance	30-Second Surges	Endurance	Even Stevens
Week 1	15 min power moves (See "Prewalk Power Moves" below.) & 25 min moderate pace walk (level 5–6) (48 min)	4 min power pace (level 7) with 2 min of moderate walking (level 5–6). Do 2 times (20 min).	15 min power moves & 25 min moderate pace walk (48 min)	30 sec sprints (level 9–10) with 1 min of easy walking (level 3–4). Do 8 times. (20 min)	15 min power moves & 25 min moderate pace walk (level 5–6) (48 min)	1 min race pace (level 8) with 1 min of moderate walking (level 5–6). Do 6 times. (20 min)
Week 2	15 min power moves & 30 min walk (53 min)	3 times (26 min)	15 min power moves & 30 min walk (53 min)	12 times (26 min)	15 min power moves & 30 min walk (53 min)	6 times, 90 sec each (26 min)
Week 3	15 min power moves & 35 min walk (58 min)	4 times (32 min)	15 min power moves & 35 min walk (58 min)	16 times (32 min)	15 min power moves & 35 min walk (58 min)	6 times, 2 min each (32 min)
Week 4	15 min power moves & 40 min walk (63 min)	4 times (32 min)	15 min power moves & 40 min walk (63 min)	16 times (32 min)	15 min power moves & 40 min walk (63 min)	6 times, 2 min each (32 min)
Week 5	15 min power moves & 45 min walk (68 min)	5 times (38 min)	15 min power moves & 45 min walk (68 min)	20 times (38 min)	15 min power moves & 45 min walk (68 min)	6 times, 2.5 min each (38 min)
Week 6	15 min power moves & 50 min walk (73 min)	5 times (38 min)	15 min power moves & 50 min walk (73 min)	20 times (38 min)	15 min power moves & 50 min walk (73 min)	6 times, 2.5 min each (38 min)

Prewalk Power Moves

Burn more fat! Although intervals are best for maximizing weight-loss, you can increase fat burn—possibly up to 15 percent—anytime you walk by strength-training before you hit the pavement, according to a Japanese study. You'll also build muscle to boost your metabolism and firm up those trouble spots. Add this 15-minute routine before your endurance walks. Do 2 sets of 10 to 15 reps of each move.

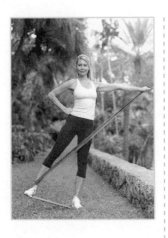

OPPOSITE ARM AND LEG PULL

WORKS SHOULDERS, HIPS, BUTT, AND OUTER THIGHS

Stand on one end of 6-foot exercise band with left foot and place right foot on band about hip-width away so band is around outside of right foot. Place right hand on hip and hold opposite end of band in left hand so it crosses body (band will be loose). Simultaneously lift right foot out to side about 45 degrees while raising left arm out to side to shoulder height. Hold for a second, then lower to start. Complete a full set, then switch sides. Do 2 sets on each side.

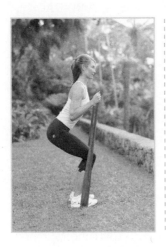

HAMMER SQUAT

WORKS ARMS, BUTT, AND THIGHS

Stand with feet shoulder-width apart, stepping on center of band. Hold ends of band in each hand so it's taut (choke up on band or wrap around hands if needed), palms facing in. Bend hips and knees and sit back as far as possible or until thighs are parallel to ground. Keep knees behind toes. At the same time, bend elbows and curl hands up toward shoulders, keeping elbows close to body. Hold for a second, then return to start.

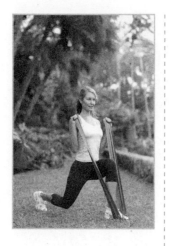

LUNGE PRESS

WORKS SHOULDERS, ARMS, BACK, ABS, BUTT, AND THIGHS

Grasp ends of band with each hand. Stand on center of band with left foot and hold ends at shoulder height, palms facing forward. Take a giant step back with right foot and bend both knees, lowering into lunge with front thigh parallel to ground. In one smooth motion, straighten left leg and press band overhead while contracting glutes and raising right leg behind you. Hold for a second, then lower back into a lunge. Complete a full set, then switch legs. Do 2 sets on each side.

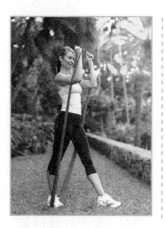

BAND FLY

WORKS SHOULDERS, CHEST, AND BACK

Stand on center of band with right foot and grasp an end in each hand. Place left foot in front of right one. Raise arms out to sides to shoulder height and bend elbows 90 degrees so arms form goalposts, palms facing forward. Squeeze chest muscles and bring forearms together in front of body. Return to start. Switch legs for a second set.

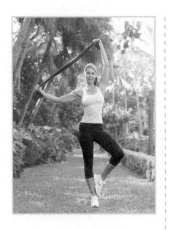

BALANCE PULLDOWN

WORKS ARMS, BACK, AND ABS

Stand with feet together. Wrap ends of band around each hand and hold it overhead with left arm above shoulder (this is anchor hand) and right arm out to side about 45 degrees. Both elbows should be slightly bent and band taut. Place sole of left foot against inside calf of right leg. Keeping left arm stable, contract ab and back muscles and pull right arm down to about shoulder height. Hold for a second, then return to start. Complete a full set, then switch arms and legs. Do 2 sets on each side.

WALK-A-MARATHON (OR HALF) PROGRAM

This customizable workout (which includes plenty of fat-burning intervals) will get you ready to achieve a fitness goal that will change your life. Join Team *Prevention* for a walking event this year. The side effects are fabulous! You'll have more energy, get fitter, slim down, boost your confidence, and make new friends.

Workout at a Glance

If you want to do a full marathon, follow the entire schedule in "Your Training Calendar" on page 183. For a half-marathon, do weeks 1 through 10, and 19 and 20. (You'll see those weeks are shaded on the schedule.) To get more training plans, go to Prevention.com/team.

The routines:

Moderate Walk (MW): Walk at a brisk pace, as if you need to get to an appointment.

Intensity Walk (IW): Walk at a brisk pace and add short bursts of speed, walking as fast as possible. Try some of the types of intervals in the Fat-Blasting Plan (see "6-Week Fat-Blasting Workout" on page 177), repeating them as needed to hit the recommended workout times in the calendar.

Cross-Train (Xtrain): To prevent burnout and injury, mix up your training by doing an activity that's different from walking, such as core workouts, weight lifting, yoga, Pilates, swimming, or cycling. Keep the intensity moderate.

Endurance Walk (EW): Walk at a slightly brisk pace, slower than a Moderate Walk but faster than a Recovery Walk. Distance, not speed, is the key here.

Recovery Walk (RW): To loosen up from the previous day's long walk, take an easy walk, strolling at a slightly faster pace than the warmup.

Always warm up by walking at a slower pace for the first 3 to 5 minutes of your workout and do the same at the end to cool down.

Running a marathon isn't for everyone, but walking may be, no matter what your fitness. Just ask some of the thousands of *Prevention* readers of all ages who've taken our annual walking challenge to lose weight, get fit, feel younger, boost their confidence, and fight disease. They say the experience changed their lives!

"Long-distance walking has helped me to be more present in my body and to be more patient," says former runner Denise Wirth, 47, who has lost 74 pounds so far.

Now it's your turn! You can choose to walk a full- or half-marathon with us and we'll be with you every step of the way, from prerace training and support to personal attention and get-togethers with *Prevention* staff at each event. With our help, you can have this life- and body-changing experience.

Team *Prevention* will be at walking events across the country this year—all of which offer full- and half-marathon options (26.2 and 13.1 miles, respectively). To register, learn more, or just get tips and train on your own for an event of your choice, go to Prevention.com/team.

HEALTH HEROES

She helped raise $30 million to bring walking paths back to her community

For decades, urban development destroyed walking and biking areas in Majora Carter's Bronx neighborhood, pushing obesity and asthma rates sky-high. Even a glimpse of the factory-lined river was impossible—she thought. "One day my puppy dragged me through a garbage field to the water's edge," says Carter, 40. "I knew that spot had to be saved." In 2001, she led local rallies to defeat plans for a nearby waste-treatment plant. She went on to found a nonprofit environmental organization called Sustainable South Bronx. Carter believes that people shouldn't have to move out of their neighborhoods to live in a better one.

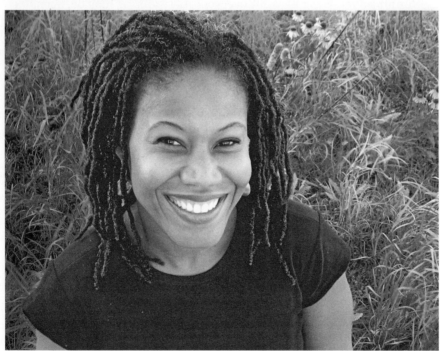

At Prevention.com/team you'll get training schedules customized just for you; top docs, dieticians, and coaches to answer your questions; weekly e-newsletters loaded with tips; mentors for extra personal guidance; and message boards to trade tips with other walkers.

YOUR TRAINING CALENDAR

	WEEK	SUNDAY	MONDAY	TUESDAY	WEDNESDAY	THURSDAY	FRIDAY	SATURDAY
ALL START	1	MW: 15 min	Xtrain: 20 min	IW: 20 min	MW: 30 min	IW: 20 min	Rest	EW: 3 miles
	2	RW: 15 min	Xtrain: 20 min	IW: 20 min	MW: 30 min	IW: 20 min	Rest	EW: 3 miles
	3	RW: 15 min	Xtrain: 20 min	IW: 20 min	MW: 30 min	IW: 20 min	Rest	EW: 4 miles
	4	RW: 15 min	Xtrain: 20 min	IW: 30 min	MW: 45 min	IW: 30 min	Rest	EW: 4 miles
	5	RW: 15 min	Xtrain: 20 min	IW: 30 min	MW: 45 min	IW: 30 min	Rest	EW: 5 miles
	6	RW: 20 min	Xtrain: 20 min	IW: 30 min	MW: 45 min	IW: 30 min	Rest	EW: 6 miles
	7	RW: 20 min	Xtrain: 20 min	IW: 45 min	MW: 60 min	IW: 45 min	Rest	EW: 6 miles
	8	RW: 20 min	Xtrain: 20 min	IW: 45 min	MW: 60 min	IW: 45 min	Rest	EW: 7 miles
HALF MARATHON TRAINS FIRST 10 WEEKS AND LAST 2 WEEKS	9	RW: 30 min	Xtrain: 20 min	IW: 45 min	MW: 60 min	IW: 45 min	Rest	EW: 8 miles
	10	RW: 30 min	Xtrain: 20 min	IW: 45 min	MW: 60 min	IW: 45 min	Rest	EW: 10 miles
	11	RW: 30 min	Xtrain: 20 min	IW: 45 min	MW: 60 min	IW: 45 min	Rest	EW: 12 miles
	12	RW: 30 min	Xtrain: 20 min	IW: 45 min	MW: 60 min	IW: 45 min	Rest	EW: 14 miles
	13	RW: 30 min	Xtrain: 20 min	IW: 60 min	MW: 90 min	IW: 60 min	Rest	EW: 7 miles
	14	RW: 30 min	Xtrain: 20 min	IW: 45 min	MW: 60 min	IW: 45 min	Rest	EW: 16 miles
	15	RW: 30 min	Xtrain: 20 min	IW: 45 min	MW: 60 min	IW: 45 min	Rest	EW: 18 miles
	16	RW: 30 min	Xtrain: 20 min	IW: 60 min	MW: 90 min	IW: 60 min	Rest	EW: 10 miles
	17	RW: 30 min	Xtrain: 20 min	IW: 45 min	MW: 60 min	IW: 45 min	Rest	EW: 20 miles
	18	RW: 30 min	Xtrain: 20 min	IW: 30 min	MW: 45 min	IW: 30 min	Rest	EW: 10 miles
FULL MARATHON TRAINS ALL WEEKS	19	RW: 30 min	Xtrain: 20 min	IW: 20 min	MW: 30 min	IW: 20 min	Rest	EW: 5 miles
	20	RW: 20 min	RW: 30 min	RW: 20 min	Rest	RW: 30 min	Rest	RW: 20 min

fast fact

54: The percentage of adults in the South Bronx who get no physical exercise at all

WIPE OUT CELLULITE

Toss the creams and dreams.
This science-proven fitness and food
plan will minimize lumps and bumps
in less than a month

Americans spend nearly $100 million on creams, lotions, and other topical treatments every year in hopes of eradicating cellulite from their thighs and butts. We're going to make a wild guess that very few of those products worked as well as you'd hoped. That's because, despite its infamy, cellulite is just plain old fat (albeit dressed up in slightly more offensive attire), and a key to minimizing it is to drop pounds, according to a study published in the journal *Plastic and Reconstructive Surgery*.

But how you lose weight matters: Crash dieting can actually make cellulite worse by reducing skin's elasticity, making more of those little puckers noticeable. Gradual weight-loss (to better preserve skin's suppleness and reduce fat) accompanied by targeted muscle development, which firms and smooths the underlying tissue, is the most effective cellulite solution, says Glynis Ablon, MD, an assistant clinical professor of dermatology at UCLA.

When Wayne Westcott, PhD, coauthor of *No More Cellulite*, tested such a strategy on 115 women, all of them reported a reduction in cellulite appearance at the end of 8 weeks, and ultrasound measurements confirmed a higher proportion of muscle to fat in their thigh areas.

Now, it's your turn. This comprehensive exercise and eating plan—designed by Chris Freytag, *Prevention*'s fitness expert and creator of *Prevention's Fight Cellulite Fast!* DVD, and based on Westcott's findings—will burn fat, build muscle, and shed pounds safely. We know it's definitely not as easy as applying a cream. But it's definately more effective. See for yourself.

THE WORKOUT

This two-pronged exercise program helps minimize the lumpy, bumpy appearance of cellulite. Aerobic exercise such as walking and running burns fat, while lower-body moves such as squats and lunges build muscle. To maximize fat loss, you will do 200 minutes of cardio a week—the amount found to produce the greatest weight-loss—including high-intensity exercise to rev your calorie burn for up to 19 hours after a workout. You should see the slimming, smoothing results in 4 weeks!

Your Plan at a Glance

This science-based, fat-blasting plan is made up of two parts. Part 1 will help you burn off cellulite. Part 2 will get you toned, smooth, and firm. We'll talk about each in turn.

Part 1: Burn Off Cellulite: You'll do this 5 days a week. Blast fat with two types of cardio routines: Intense Workouts (an interval program that builds from fitness walks to calorie-blasting runs) and Moderate Workouts (any aerobic activity you enjoy).

	INTENSE WORKOUTS: 3 DAYS A WEEK				MODERATE WORKOUTS: 2 DAYS A WEEK
Week	Brisk Walk interval	Run interval*	Number of intervals	Total workout (5 min warmup, 5 min cooldown included)	You choose: walking, swimming, or cycling
1	2 min	1 min	10	40 min	40 min
2	1 min	1 min	15	40 min	40 min
3	1 min	2 min	10	40 min	40 min
4	1 min	4 min	7	45 min	40 min
5	1 min	6 min	5	45 min	40 min
6	1 min	7 min	4	42 min	40 min
7	1 min	8 min	4	46 min	40 min
8	1 min	9 min	3	40 min	40 min

*If you have joint problems, you can substitute fast walking for running.

Part 2: Tone, Smooth, and Firm: You'll do this 3 days a week. Tone your muscles by doing the six strengthening moves shown on the following pages. (Take a day off between these workouts.)

Weeks 1 and 2: Do 1 set of 12 repetitions of each exercise.

Weeks 3 and 4: Repeat the circuit twice so you're doing 2 sets of each exercise.

Weeks 5 through 8: Repeat the circuit 3 times, so you're doing 3 sets of each exercise. But on the third set, instead of holding each move, try to pulse for 3 counts by lifting and lowering a few inches before returning to the start position.

These six moves tone your hips, butt, and thighs, which are the most common sites for cellulite. For each move we offer an easier option, in case the main move is too difficult. If it's too easy, increase the intensity of the standing exercises by holding dumbbells. To avoid injury, warm up with 5 minutes of marching in place or do these moves directly after your cardio workout when muscles are already warmed.

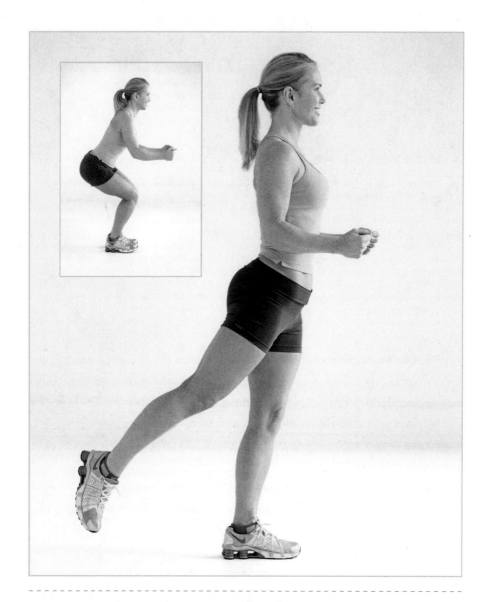

SQUAT KICKBACK

Stand with feet together, toes pointing forward, and arms bent at sides. Bend knees and hips into a squat, as if you were sitting in a chair, and hold for 3 counts. As you rise, press right leg back and squeeze glutes. Hold for 1 count, then lower. Switch legs after each set.

Make it easier: Don't squat as deeply, and keep toes on floor when pressing back.

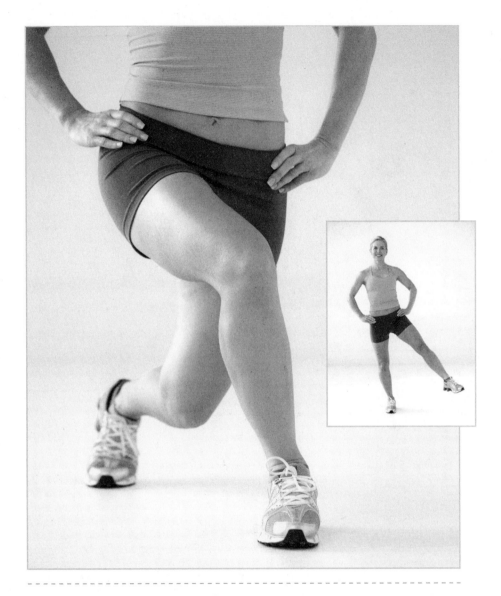

CURTSY AND KICK

Stand with feet together, hands on hips. Step left foot behind right leg and bend knees until right thigh is almost parallel to floor. Keep right knee over ankle. Hold for 3 counts. As you stand back up, kick left leg out to side before doing another curtsy. Switch legs after each set.

Make it easier: Skip the kick and bring feet together between each curtsy.

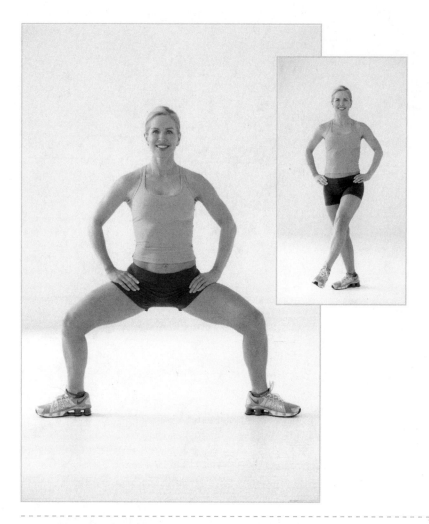

PLIÉ SWEEP

Stand with feet wide apart, toes pointing out, and hands on hips. Keeping back straight and abs tight, tuck tailbone and bend knees, lowering until thighs are almost parallel to floor. Hold for 3 counts. As you stand up, sweep left leg across body, as if you're kicking a soccer ball. Switch legs after each set.

Make it easier: Eliminate the leg sweep.

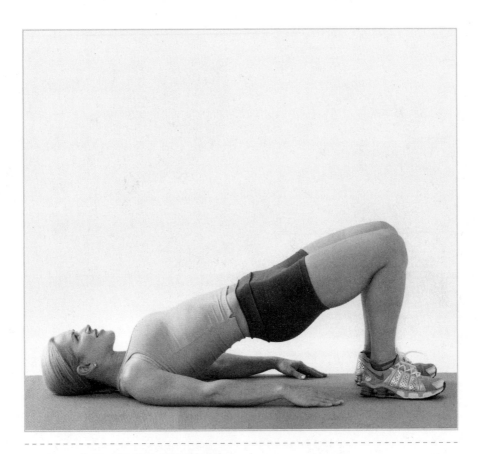

GLUTE SQUEEZE

Lie on floor with knees bent, feet beneath knees and hip-width apart. Keeping hips level and abs tight, press into heels and squeeze glutes, lifting hips to form a bridge. Lower hips halfway to floor for 2 counts, then press back up. (Instead of pulses on your third set, do a Hip Rock: In bridge position, squeeze left buttocks and lift left hip. Repeat on right side. That's 1 rep.)

Make it easier: Lower hips to floor between reps.

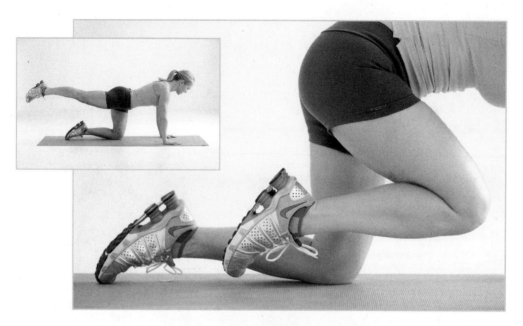

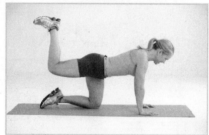

BUN BURNER

Get on all fours, with hands beneath shoulders, knees beneath hips, and abs tight. Extend right leg behind you so it's in line with back, toes pointed and hips square to floor. Pull knee into chest, contracting abs, and extend leg back out 12 times. Next, extend right leg and pulse, lifting and lowering a few inches, 12 times. Then bend right leg so sole of foot faces ceiling and pulse 12 times. That's 1 set. Repeat with left leg. (No need to add additional pulses when you progress to 3 sets.)

Make it easier: Place forearms on floor.

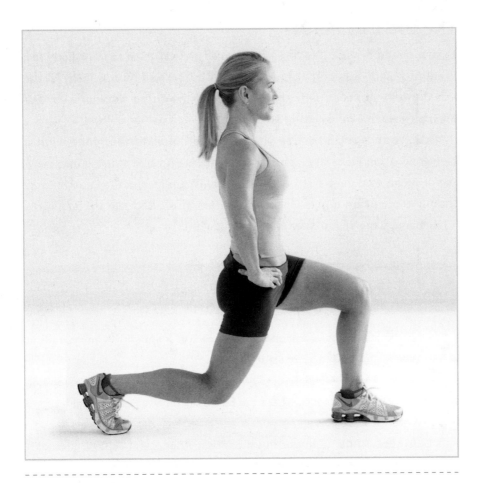

PASS-THROUGH LUNGES

Stand with feet together, hands on hips. Step left foot forward 2 to 3 feet and bend knees, lowering until left thigh is parallel to floor. Keep left knee over ankle. Hold for 1 count. In one swift movement, press off left foot and bring it behind you. (Right foot doesn't move.) Lower into another lunge so right thigh is parallel to floor, holding for 1 count. Continue passing left foot through into a front then a back lunge without bringing feet together. Switch legs after each set.

Make it easier: Rather than pushing through from front to back in one swift movement, bring feet together before going into back lunge.

THE EATING PLAN

Lose a pound a week. Maybe two. That's the best pace to shed body fat; gradual weight-loss may help smooth out lumps and bumps. Stay in the slow lane—and keep fueling your cellulite-smoothing workouts—by following these five fat-blasting strategies.

Cue your portions. Use your hand to help you recognize what a healthy portion looks like. Your palm is about the size of a 3-ounce serving of meat, and your fist is good for a half cup, perfect for pasta. Your thumb is about an ounce (cheese is 1½ thumbs), and the tip measures 1 teaspoon, which counts for one serving of oil.

FOODS THAT FIGHT FAT

Add these items to your shopping list to curb your appetite, burn fat, and put you on the road to a smoother you.

OATMEAL: A study found that the fiber in the rolled grain curbs your appetite without a truckload of calories. That's the perfect combo to help you eat less and lose weight.

VEGETABLE JUICE: Consider this a calorie-cutting cocktail: One glass of it before mealtime, and you'll eat up to 135 fewer calories later, according to scientists at Pennsylvania State University.

NUTS: Add a few small servings of your favorite variety to your diet. The fiber and good fat in nuts makes them very filling, so your weight stays steady, say researchers at Loma Linda University.

FAT-FREE MILK: Several studies have shown a link between calcium and body fat: As calcium intake increases, body fat decreases. And one study showed that two servings of dairy every day may reduce the risk of gaining weight by as much as 70 percent.

GREEN TEA: Compounds in this type of tea may help boost your body's metabolism and fat-burning abilities, according to double-blind, controlled clinical studies.

Graze, don't gorge. Plan on three small meals and two or three snacks a day, spaced no more than 4 hours apart. People who followed this mini-meal plan were leaner and had less body fat than people who ate the same number of calories packed into two or three big meals, found researchers at the University of Michigan. Eating small portions often also helps keep your metabolism revved and stomach full so you don't overeat.

Cut 100 calories per meal. It's a lot easier than you may think, and it adds up fast: With 300 to 500 calories cut plus 400 more burned with our exercise plan, you'll lose slow and steady. Skip the croutons in your salad and use 1 less tablespoon of butter on bread; both are good for saving 100 calories. For more ideas, visit Prevention.com/100calories.

Choose extra-filling foods. That means those that are high in fiber and water, such as broth-based soups and raw veggies, which are particularly talented at quelling appetite, so you'll want to stop eating sooner. A study of 150 overweight people found that those who ate soup every day for a year lost 50 percent more weight than people who didn't. And munching on a salad with fat-free dressing before your meal may cut your calorie intake by 12 percent, according to another study.

Pass on processed junk. Cookies, crackers, chips, and more—they're all packed with a lot of calories and not nearly enough nutrients per ounce as healthier options. A Centers for Disease Control and Prevention survey of more than 7,000 adults confirmed that women who ate a calorie-dense diet had a higher BMI and weighed more.

GET A METABOLISM THAT SOARS

Our fat-fighting diet and exercise plan will help you drop major pounds at any age

You probably don't need scientists to tell you that your metabolism slows with age. But they're studying it anyway—and coming up with exciting new research to help rev it up again. The average woman gains 1½ pounds a year during her adult life—enough to pack on 40-plus pounds by her fifties if she doesn't combat the roller coaster of hormones, muscle loss, and stress that conspires to slow her fat-burning engine.

We've found a plan that will tackle all these. *Prevention*'s customizable metabolism-boosting routine will help you shed up to 8 pounds in just 4 weeks. Most important, you'll have a lean, strong physique and energy to spare—for life.

Our plan was created by an all-star team. Joy Prouty, an American College of Sports Medicine–certified fitness director and cocreator of the *Fit Over 50* DVD series, designed the workout. Dan Benardot, PhD, RD, an associate professor of nutrition and kinesiology at Georgia State University, and Tammy Lakatos, RD, coauthor of *Fire Up Your Metabolism*, designed the diet.

At the heart of the plan is the High-Metabolism Workout, five super-effective strength moves that build firm, lean muscle tissue, which is the key to a robust metabolism. Muscle burns up to seven times as many calories at rest as fat does, so the more muscle you have, the higher your metabolism. That's just the beginning. Each stage of your life presents special metabolism-slowing risks, including disrupted sleep and even seismic hormone shifts. So we have included a decade-by-decade, fat-fighting prescription guaranteed to keep your metabolism in high gear. And to really make it soar, there's also a High-Metabolism Diet. Start today, and you'll sleep better, have more energy, feel firmer, and notice your clothes are looser in as little as 2 weeks.

YOUR 3-STEP METABOLISM MAKEOVER

Do the High-Metabolism Workout exercise beginning on page 200 to firm up and build muscle. Everyone should do this routine 2 or 3 nonconsecutive days a week.

Add the appropriate Bonus Moves and Bigger Boost cardio prescriptions based on your age for an extra metabolism jolt.

Follow the High-Metabolism Diet advice (see page 208) to crank up your calorie burn throughout the day.

HIGH-METABOLISM WORKOUT

Strength training builds calorie-blasting muscle, which halts the 15 to 20 percent drop in your resting metabolism (the daily amount of calories you use just living and breathing) that can occur as you get older, and can boost your calorie burn by up to 10 percent. Research also shows that lifting weights just twice a week can specifically reverse age-related decline in the function of mitochondria, which are the cellular powerhouses that fuel muscles to use more oxygen and zap more calories.

Workout at a Glance

What you need: An exercise mat and two sets of dumbbells, a heavy pair (about 10 to 15 pounds) and a lighter pair (5 to 8 pounds).

How to do it: Perform this workout on 2 or 3 nonconsecutive days a week, adding Bonus Moves and Bigger Boost cardio routines as prescribed for your age. Do 2 sets of each exercise. One day, use the heavier weights for 8 to 10 reps per set. The next, do 12 to 14 reps per set with the lighter dumbbells.

REFUEL, GUILT FREE

A postworkout snack can undo all of your hard work. Refuel without eating back all the calories you burned with these tips from Indiana University researcher Joel Stager, PhD.

YOU DO	BEST POST-EXERCISE SNACK
30-minute walk	A glass of water
Cardio intervals (45 minutes)	A 100-calorie snack, such as a cup of fat-free yogurt and a handful of Cheerios
6-mile power walk (about 90 minutes)	A 150-calorie snack, such as half of a PB&J sandwich (light on the peanut butter)
1 hour of strength training	A regular meal within half an hour of finishing your session

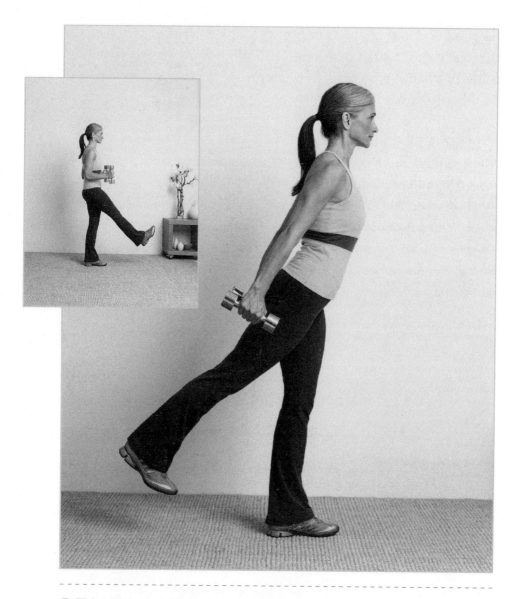

PENDULUM KICKBACK

TONES TRICEPS, BUTT, AND THIGHS

Holding a dumbbell in each hand, stand with right leg straight in front of you, 6 to 12 inches off floor, foot flexed, and elbows bent 90 degrees so forearms are parallel to floor. Swing right leg behind you, and squeeze glutes as you straighten arms. Return to start. Repeat for a full set; switch legs.

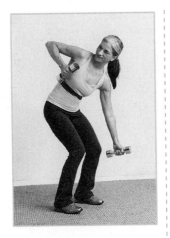

CROUCH & PULL

TONES SHOULDERS, UPPER BACK, ARMS, OBLIQUES, BUTT, AND THIGHS

Stand with feet about shoulder-width apart and sit back into partial squat. Hold a weight in each hand and hinge forward from hips about 45 degrees, arms below shoulders, palms facing in. Keeping lower body still, rotate torso to right, bend right arm, and pull dumbbell toward chest, elbow pointing toward ceiling. Return to start; repeat, alternating sides. (If you have back problems, use one weight at a time and place other hand on a chair for support.)

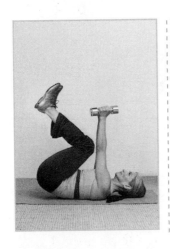

KNEE-HUGGER CHEST FLY

TONES CHEST AND ABS

Holding dumbbells in hands, lie faceup with knees bent, shins parallel to floor, arms out to sides, elbows slightly bent, and palms facing ceiling. Contract abs and lift hips about 3 inches off floor. At the same time, squeeze chest muscles and raise arms, bringing dumbbells together over chest. Lower to start and repeat.

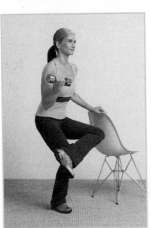

FIGURE-4 SQUAT CURL

TONES BICEPS, BUTT, AND THIGHS

Hold a dumbbell in right hand at side, palm forward. Cross left ankle over right thigh (hold a chair if needed). Bend right knee and hips, sitting back (keep knee behind toes) as you raise weight to right shoulder. Return to start. Repeat for a full set; switch sides.

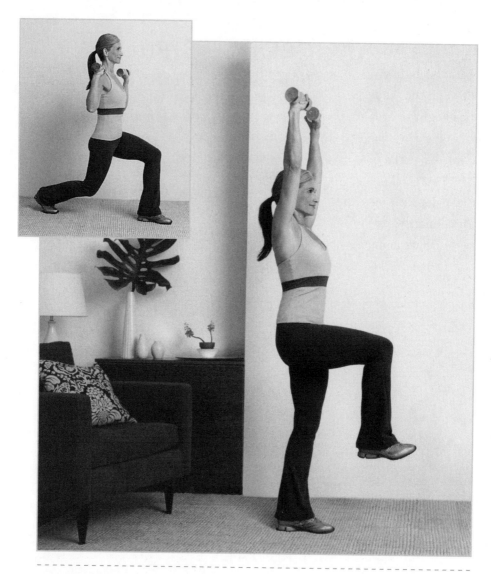

LIFTOFF LUNGE

TONES SHOULDERS, TRICEPS, BUTT, AND THIGHS

Stand with feet hip-width apart, dumbbells at shoulders, palms forward. Step right foot back about 2 feet, bend both knees, and lower until left thigh is about parallel to floor, knee over ankle. Press into left foot and stand up as you pull right knee forward (so you're balancing on left leg), and press weights overhead. Without touching floor, swing right leg back into lunge position as you lower weights. Repeat for a full set; switch legs.

BONUS MOVES FOR YOUR FORTIES

Add the following yoga moves either after work or before bed. Flow through the sequence three times. As you enter perimenopause, your ovaries begin to produce less estrogen, and the side effects—primarily disrupted sleep—can slow your metabolism. Yoga, and the deep breathing it requires, is the perfect antidote because it lowers levels of the stress hormone cortisol, reduces hot flashes, and helps you sleep more soundly. Sleep deprivation affects hormones such as leptin and ghrelin, which regulate energy expenditure, according to a Stanford University study. The researchers found that body weight rose proportionately as hours of shut-eye dropped below about 7½ a night.

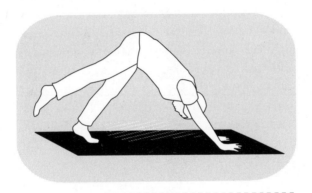

WAGGING DOWNWARD DOG

TONES SHOULDERS, BACK, BUTT, AND THIGHS

Begin on hands and knees, with hands shoulder-width apart, feet hip-width apart, toes tucked under. Press into palms, straighten legs, and lift tailbone toward ceiling, pulling navel toward spine. Raise right leg and circle it clockwise three times, making circles as large as possible without moving the rest of body. Reverse direction and repeat. Switch legs, repeat, and then lower back to floor.

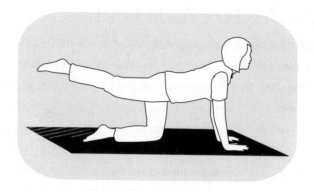

SUNBIRD

TONES BACK, ABS, AND GLUTES

Begin on hands and knees, hands directly beneath shoulders, knees directly beneath hips, and head in line with spine. Tuck chin toward chest and draw right knee toward forehead. Lift head to look up, while extending right leg behind you as high as possible without overarching back, toes pointed. Hold for 5 seconds, then pull knee back in. Do five times, then switch legs.

For a Bigger Boost

Do mini cardio workouts. Aim for three 10- to 15-minute bouts throughout the day, at least 5 days a week. At this stage, you're probably already juggling the demands of growing children, aging parents, and a career. Mini-workouts are your best bet for fitting in exercise, and they may even rev up your fat burn better. In one study, women who exercised for 10 minutes three times a day lost 30 percent more fat than those who did one longer workout daily.

BONUS MOVES FOR YOUR FIFTIES

Add the following exercises to your High-Metabolism Workout, performing the same number of sets and reps as outlined in that routine. As you approach menopause, estrogen levels decline dramatically, making fat cells your body's primary source of estrogen, says Harvard Medical School researcher JoAnn Manson, MD, author of *Hot Flashes, Hormones & Your Health*. At the same time, levels of growth hormones important for muscle building also decline. The combination sets you up to gain more fat and lose more muscle, but you can counteract these changes with some extra strength training. It's the best way to rev up your metabolism and may boost hormone levels.

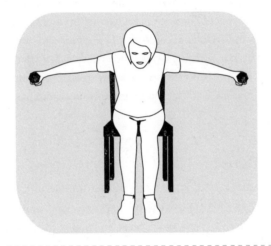

SEATED BACK FLY

TONES SHOULDERS AND UPPER BACK

Holding dumbbells, sit on chair with feet flat on floor. Keeping back straight, lean forward from hips about 45 degrees so arms hang toward floor, palms facing in. Squeeze shoulder blades together and raise arms out to sides (don't lock elbows) until parallel to floor. Lower and repeat.

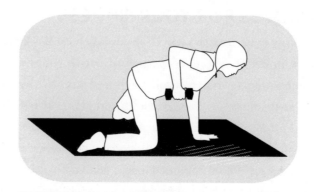

TRIPOD ROW

TONES BACK AND ARMS

Kneel on floor holding dumbbell in right hand. Place both hands on floor directly beneath shoulders, right knee directly beneath hip, and extend left leg out to side, foot flexed and inside of foot on floor. Keeping head in line with back, bend right elbow and pull dumbbell to ribs, elbow pointing toward ceiling. Lower and repeat. Complete a set; switch sides.

For a Bigger Boost

Do cardio intervals. Add four to six 30- to 60-second bursts of vigorous activity (speed walking, running, or jumping rope) to your usual cardio routine two or three times a week. "My research shows that exercising at high-intensity efforts raises your metabolism enough to stay elevated several hours after your workout," says William Kraemer, PhD, a professor of kinesiology, physiology, neurobiology, and medicine at the University of Connecticut. "This can add up to 50 calories or more."

BONUS MOVES FOR YOUR SIXTIES

Add the following exercises to your High-Metabolism Workout, performing the same number of sets and reps as outlined in that routine. Researchers at the University of Maryland found that after menopause, women lost nearly six times as much muscle mass and were half as active in their leisure time as their premenopausal peers. As a result, their resting metabolism fell by more than 100 calories a day, compared with a mere 8-calorie decline among premenopausal women. Core exercises best combat that accelerated muscle loss and prevent the aches that discourage you from moving. "The muscles in your back and abdominals literally hold you up and give you strength from the inside out, so you can be more active with less aches and pains," says Prouty. And you'll stand taller, instead of hunching forward, and build more muscle.

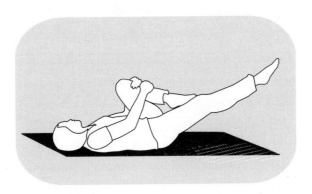

SINGLE-LEG STRETCH

TONES ABS AND THIGHS

Lie on back with knees bent, shins parallel to floor. Tilt pelvis to flatten back to floor. Keeping abs tight, extend right leg to a 45-degree angle with floor and pull left knee to chest, grasping shin with both hands. Switch legs. Repeat, alternating legs for 20 total reps. For a greater challenge, keep head and shoulders lifted off floor as you do reps.

(continued on page 210)

HIGH-METABOLISM DIET

The following essential eating rules stoke your fat burn all day long.

EAT ENOUGH. You need to cut calories to lose weight. But going too low is bad. When you eat less than you need for basic biological function (about 1,200 calories for most women), your body throws the brakes on your metabolism.

It also begins to break down precious, calorie-burning muscle tissue for energy, says Dan Benardot, PhD, RD, an associate professor of nutrition and kinesiology at Georgia State University. "Eat just enough so you're not hungry—a 150-calorie snack midmorning and midafternoon between three meals (about 430 calories each) will keep your metabolism humming."

REV UP IN THE MORNING. Eating breakfast jump-starts metabolism and keeps energy high all day. It's no accident that women who skip this meal are four and a half times as likely to be obese. If nothing else, grab a yogurt. Or try oatmeal made with fat-free milk and topped with nuts for an essential protein boost.

DRINK COFFEE OR TEA. Caffeine is a central nervous system stimulant, so your daily java jolts can rev up your metabolism 5 to 8 percent—about 98 to 174 calories a day. A cup of brewed tea can raise your metabolism by 12 percent, according to one Japanese study. Researchers believe the antioxidant catechin in tea provides the boost.

FIGHT FAT WITH FIBER. Research shows that some fiber can rev up your fat burn by as much as 30 percent. (To learn more, see chapter 15.) Studies find that women who eat the most fiber gain the least weight over time. Aim for about 25 grams a day—the amount in about three servings each of fruits and vegetables.

BUY THE BIG BOTTLE. German researchers found that drinking 6 cups of cold water a day (that's 48 ounces) can raise resting metabolism by about 50 calories daily. That's enough to shed 5 pounds in a year. The increase may come from the work it takes to heat the water to body temperature.

GO ORGANIC. Canadian researchers report that dieters with the most organochlorines (pollutants from pesticides, which are stored in fat cells) experience a greater-than-normal dip in metabolism as they lose weight, perhaps because the toxins interfere with the energy-burning process. Other research hints that pesticides can trigger weight gain.

Always choose organic when buying peaches, apples, bell peppers, celery, nectarines, potatoes, spinach, strawberries, cherries, lettuce, imported grapes, and pears. They tend to have the highest levels of pesticides.

ALWAYS INCLUDE PROTEIN. Your body needs protein to maintain lean muscle. Add a serving, such as 3 ounces of lean meat, 2 tablespoons of nuts, or 8 ounces of low-fat yogurt, to every meal and snack. Research shows protein can increase postmeal calorie burn by as much as 35 percent.

EAT IRON-RICH FOODS. It's essential for carrying the oxygen your muscles need to burn fat, says Tammy Lakatos, RD, coauthor of *Fire Up Your Metabolism*. Until menopause, women lose iron each month through menstruation. Unless you restock your stores, you run the risk of low energy and a sagging metabolism. Shellfish, lean meats, beans, fortified cereals, and spinach are excellent sources.

GET MORE D. This vitamin is essential for preserving metabolism-revving muscle tissue. Unfortunately, researchers estimate that a measly 4 percent of Americans over age 50 take in enough through their diet. Get 90 percent of your recommended daily value (400 IU) in a 3.5-ounce serving of salmon. Other good sources: tuna, shrimp, tofu, fortified milk and cereal, and eggs.

SKIP THE SECOND COCKTAIL. When you have a drink, you burn less fat, and more slowly than usual, because the alcohol is used as fuel instead. Knocking back two martinis can reduce your body's fat-burning ability by up to 73 percent.

DRINK MILK. "There's some evidence that calcium deficiency, which is common in many women, may slow metabolism," says Lakatos. Research shows that consuming calcium through dairy foods such as fat-free milk and low-fat yogurt may also reduce fat absorption from other foods.

FIDGET. Regular daily activity known as "NEAT" (nonexercise activity thermogenesis) is essential for a healthy metabolism. Small movements such as stretching your legs, taking the stairs, even just standing to talk on the phone can add up to an extra 350 calories burned a day. (For more NEAT moves, see chapter 24.)

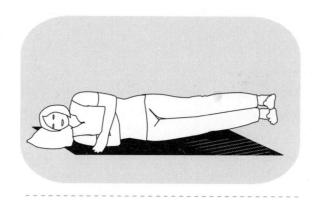

SIDE LEG LIFT

TONES SIDES OF TORSO, BACK AND THIGHS

Lie on right side, arms crossed over chest (place pillow or towel under head for support, if needed), legs extended, feet flexed and stacked. Contract abs and back and lift both legs 2 to 4 inches off floor, then lower. Do 10 reps, switch sides, and repeat.

For a Bigger Boost

Do longer cardio sessions. Increase these workouts to 45 to 50 minutes, 5 days a week. A University of Colorado study of 65 women found that postmenopausal women who did so maintained the same resting metabolic rate as their younger, premenopausal peers. "Activities that engage both your upper and lower body, such as walking with poles, are especially good calorie burners, and they help keep those upper-body muscles strong and extra firm as well," says Prouty.

MOVE IT TO LOSE IT

Research shows that the little stuff you do all day can add up to big weight-loss. Five readers put that theory to the test, with "wow" results

To lose pounds and keep them off, burning calories is key. Not just at the gym; being active throughout the day can add up to big weight-loss, too. James Levine, MD, of the Mayo Clinic in Rochester, Minnesota, has spent a decade studying the role that every movement, or nonexercise activity thermogenesis (NEAT), plays in metabolism. His discovery: People who tap their feet, prefer standing to sitting, and generally move a lot burn up to 350 more calories a day than those who sit still. That adds up to nearly 37 pounds a year!

Prevention fitness expert Chris Freytag has come up with a dozen ways to increase your NEAT level and add short bursts of exercise to your day to amplify your calorie burn. We had five busy women road test the tips while they were wearing a calorie-counting bodybugg armband ($300; bodybugg.com). The results: They burned as many as 500 extra calories a day—without breaking a sweat—and lost up to 7 pounds during our 2-week test. Here's how they did it, and how you can, too!

fast fact

Brief bursts of intense exercise can provide the same cardiovascular benefits as long-term exercise. Researchers at McMaster University found that 6 weeks of interval training using 30-second sprints three times a week improves the cardiovascular arteries just as much as 40 to 60 minutes of cycling five times a week.

DO CRUNCHES IN BED

Calorie burn: Up to 20 calories in less than 5 minutes

Get a jump-start on flatter abs before your feet even hit the floor, says Freytag. Simply draw your knees toward your chest 25 to 50 times to rev up your energy, tone your belly, and burn 15 to 20 calories. Add a set at night to double your burn.

DANCE WHILE YOU DRESS

Calorie burn: Up to 55 calories in about an hour

When tester Lesa Kennedy flipped on her favorite R&B station, she burned 55 extra calories as she got dressed and packed lunch. "The beat inspired me to add shakes and shimmies to my usual routine. My daughter loved it, and we started our day off in a great mood," she says.

CIRCLE THE BLOCK

Calorie burn: Up to 375 calories throughout the day

Research shows that the more comfortable your clothes, the more active you'll be throughout the day. Make it a rule to wear shoes comfy enough for a 5-mile walk, and look for ways to add bits of strolling all day long. Lap the grocery store before you pick up your first item or take a 15-minute midday walk.

"At work I take the stairs to use a bathroom on a different floor," says tester Elizabeth Lissmann.

STAND UP MORE

Calorie burn: Up to 200 calories in about an hour

With their jam-packed days, our testers are no strangers to multitasking. But Freytag found that they could boost their metabolism simply by spending more time on their feet. Rather than sitting on a bench while her children played at the park, for example, tester Melissa Fitzgerald walked around the playground area for 15 minutes and melted 50 extra calories.

Kennedy torched 120 more calories in an hour by standing during her daughter's dance class. "All the other moms repeatedly offered me a seat," she says. "They couldn't understand why I wanted to stand!"

TAKE A COMEDY BREAK

Calorie burn: Up to 40 calories in about 15 minutes

Research shows that laughing for 10 to 15 minutes (such as when watching a funny half-hour sitcom) can burn about 40 calories. It's a small number by itself, says Freytag, but a daily chuckle could add up to a loss of about 4 pounds over a year. That motivated Lissmann to look for humor throughout the day, such as watching comedy sketches on YouTube during a lunch break.

PLAY THE POST-IT GAME

Calorie burn: Up to 240 calories throughout the day

Get your kids in on the fun with this fitness scavenger hunt that helped Kennedy burn an extra 240 calories on a Saturday afternoon. Write exercises on five or six sticky notes—50 jumping jacks, 20 crunches, 10 pushups, and 25 lunges, for example—and give them to your children to hide in the house. When you discover a note, follow the instructions, then look for the next one.

TARGET ONE BODY PART A DAY

Calorie burn: Up to 50 calories in 10 minutes

Fitzgerald often set a big goal—such as working out for an hour—and when that wasn't possible she ended up doing nothing. Instead, Freytag suggested focusing on one body part daily for 10 minutes. Fitzgerald sneaked in mini-workouts—without even changing clothes—while her boys were watching a video. She did lunges and squats one day followed by situps and bench dips the next day. "It gave me extra energy, so rather than lying on the sofa at night, I'd clean the kitchen and burn even more calories," she says.

MAKE MULTIPLE TRIPS

Calorie burn: Up to 80 calories throughout the day

When there's laundry or groceries to bring upstairs, people have the tendency to pile as much as possible in their arms and make one trip, says Freytag, but they're missing a great opportunity for exercise. Carry each bag or item one at a time. Or try Lissmann's trick: "Instead of waiting until I have a big pile of documents to fax, I send each one as it's ready. The faxes get out faster and I add extra steps to my day!"

MEET THE TESTERS

These five *Prevention* readers put to the test the theory that the little movements you do all day can add up to big weight loss.

KATE RIVAS, 50, burned 500 extra calories a day!

Before: I gained 35 pounds after taking a job that keeps me chained to my desk for hours at a time.

After: I put a Gaiam Mini-Stepper ($69; amazon.com) under my desk. Now when I'm on the phone I can pedal away calories. I lost 7 pounds in 2 weeks!

MELISSA FITZGERALD, 40, burned 200 extra calories a day!

Before: I used to be a runner, but with two boys under age 6 I struggle to fit exercise into my list of priorities.

After: I run alongside my kids when they're riding their bikes, and I have more energy now!

ELIZABETH LISSMANN, 47, burned 240 extra calories a day!

Before: My asthma makes it tough to complete a full-blown workout, so I hate going to the gym.

After: I learned that I can string together a series of small events that will create one big workout. For example, if I stand up and walk for 5 minutes every hour, at the end of the day I've walked at least 50 to 60 minutes.

LESA KENNEDY, 45, burned 312 extra calories a day!

Before: Between my desk job, shuttling my child to school and activities, taking care of my elderly mom, and attending night school, I sit for 8 to 10 hours a day.

After: Instead of waiting in front of the microwave for my food to cook, I take a lap around the office. I've lost an inch off my hips!

STEPHANIE CARROLL, 45, burned 208 extra calories a day!

Before: I was skeptical that these small changes would make a difference.

After: Now if my kids want something from another floor, I don't mind running to get it. I lost 2 pounds during the 2-week test.

FIDGET (FREQUENTLY!)

Calorie burn: Up to 350 calories throughout the day

Dr. Levine's research shows that fidgeting can add up to 350 calories a day. "I had to make a conscious effort by posting a reminder on my desk," says Kennedy, "but once I started trying things like pacing while I talked on the phone, bouncing my knee at my desk, or shifting in my seat, I became more aware of how every movement burns calories."

MOVE TO TV MUSIC

Calorie burn: Up to 220 calories in half an hour

Enjoy your show while being active. "I was up during the ads for *Dancing with the Stars* and when the program came back on, I kept right on moving with the music," says tester Kate Rivas. Poof, another 110 calories gone in 15 minutes. Use commercials as exercise breaks, too: Rotate between jumping jacks, situps, pushups, and jogging in place, changing activities with each new ad (about every 30 seconds). "I burned nearly an extra 90 calories during my favorite hour-long show," says tester Stephanie Carroll.

CHAPTER 25

FINISH FEELING FABULOUS, NOT FATIGUED

How to prolong your workout afterglow

You know exercise makes you feel *good*. (A workout at the gym or a walk outside in the fresh air can help calm you down. Plus, exercise stimulates brain chemicals, which can make you feel happier.) But is feeling *good* good enough? Why not feel *great*?

Harnessing—and maximizing—the restorative powers of your workout can send your mood soaring and get you psyched for tomorrow's session. *Prevention* pored over the research and consulted experts, including PhDs and even a hypnotist. We found the following easy, effective strategies to keep you revved long after you've unlaced your walking shoes.

DRINK CAFFEINE

This stimulant doesn't just give you the energy to start your workout: Research suggests that it may help you feel better once you're done, too. Women who consumed the equivalent of 2½ cups of coffee an hour before a 30-minute bike ride reduced leg muscle pain by nearly half, compared with those who didn't have caffeine, according to a study published in *Medicine & Science in Sports & Exercise*. Caffeine appears to work on the inflammatory agent known as adenosine.

"It may block the chemical from binding to brain or muscle receptors associated with pain," says lead researcher Robert Motl, PhD, an assistant professor of kinesiology and community health at the University of Illinois at Urbana–Champaign. Even just a cup of joe might add some oomph to your moves while easing pain.

USE YOUR NOSE

Stimulating scents wake up your brain and body, suggests a study at Wheeling Jesuit University. Athletes who walked on a treadmill for 15 minutes while inhaling a peppermint aroma felt more invigorated afterward than those who walked without smelling anything.

"Peppermint increases brain activity in areas that heighten alertness," says lead researcher Bryan Raudenbush, PhD, an associate professor of psychology. The rejuvenating scent can also help enhance your workout so you experience that natural high faster. Although sniffing peppermint produces the best results, you can get a boost from flavored gums, mints, or a beverage such as Metromint water.

Another feel-good fragrance? Jasmine. Raudenbush says inhaling the sweet aroma after exercise helps your heart rate and blood pressure return to normal more quickly as you cool down, allowing your body to recuperate faster from a tough workout.

BREATHE DEEPLY

Oxygen-rich blood keeps your heart, lungs, and muscles operating at optimal efficiency so you feel fired up—not drained—during and after exercise. A great way to maximize oxygen flow is with tai chi, which is a Chinese system of exercise that emphasizes deep breathing from the abdomen.

A BRIGHTER WORKOUT

Some trainers swear that each color—part of the spectrum of light, or energy—can affect your workout. Experts are just now studying this one, but it can't hurt to slip on a bright sports tank. Red is thought to boost heart rate and energy, says Christina Leon, creator of the Colorgize fitness method, which incorporates color and lights into gym classes.

"Focusing your breath this way enhances lung capacity, and the subsequent increase in oxygen boosts energy," says Ron Knaus, DO, author of *A B Chi*.

Try tai chi breathing between strength-training sets: Standing tall with feet hip-width apart and arms at sides, take a deep breath into your belly as you clench your fists and raise both of your arms out to the sides and overhead. Relax your hands, lightly touching your thumbs and forefingers, and slowly exhale as you lower your arms back to the start. Repeat 10 times.

TAKE THE RIGHT VITAMINS

Two-thirds of adult women don't get enough iron, which is an oversight that saps energy. We need this mineral to make hemoglobin, the red-blood-cell protein that carries oxygen throughout the body.

"The deficiency is more common in active people because the body loses iron and other minerals through sweat," says Leslie Bonci, RD, director of sports nutrition at the University of Pittsburgh. Adult women need 18 milligrams of iron a day. (Women need only 8 milligrams after menopause.) Get it from red meat (2 to 3 milligrams per 3-ounce serving of cooked lean beef), fortified cereals, or a multivitamin.

Low zinc levels can also leave you dragging. Exercisers who didn't meet their daily requirement had less efficient heart rates and more trou-

DOUBLE YOUR BLISS

Sticking to a fitness routine over time can double its mood-boosting power, finds a Sacramento, California, VA Medical Center study. While nonexercisers felt happier and less stressed after a single session, adults who worked out three times a week for 6 months got those perks plus a bigger energy boost, improving their mood even more.

ble breathing during exercise, found a study in the *American Journal of Clinical Nutrition.*

"Besides helping to make muscle, zinc regulates hormones that allow our bodies to access stored energy," says study author Henry Lukaski, PhD. Poultry and beans are good sources for getting the 8 milligrams you need a day.

HYDRATE EARLY

"Dehydration depletes the body of the nourishment it needs to function at its peak," says Bonci. To boost performance, load up on liquids before you start sweating. "Sip 20 ounces of water an hour before exercise to give it time to circulate throughout your body," she says. To maintain good hydration during your workout, shoot for 14 ounces of fluid per hour if you don't sweat a lot, and 20 ounces per hour if you're the type who ends up dripping.

PICTURE VICTORY

Visualizing success while exercising can actually make your physical workout feel easier and more rewarding. Skyler Madison, a hypnotist and yoga instructor in New York City, recommends focusing on what you're achieving rather than letting your mind wander to your to-do list, which can trigger feelings of annoyance and stress.

Playing a mental image in your head—seeing your goal weight on your scale or zipping up a pair of perfectly fitting jeans—enhances positive feelings. Then, after your workout, sit or lie quietly and meditate on the good you've done for yourself and your body, the progress you're making toward your goals, and how proud you are of your accomplishments. No matter how tough the session you just completed, this practice teaches you to associate your workout with the afterglow of success.

Just say ahh.

PART

V

MIND
MATTERS

GET SMARTER

Figure out your naturally sharpest moments, and do everything a little easier, quicker, and better

Your energy level isn't the only thing about your body that varies over the course of the day. Your brain obeys its own rhythm, too—based largely on your sleep pattern, exposure to light, and genetic makeup—and getting in a groove with its tempo can make you healthier, happier, and more productive. For example: Because adults over 40 are generally morning types, they would most likely score better on an IQ test at 9 a.m. than at 4 p.m., says Lynn Hasher, PhD, a psychology professor at the University of Toronto.

As cutting-edge research by Hasher and other brain experts shows, you can burn more calories from exercise, work more efficiently, and even have better sex by learning how to sync up to your brain's power hours. Here's your daily guide.

7 TO 9 A.M.

Prime time for: Passion

"The perfect moment for bonding with your spouse is right when you wake up," says Ilia Karatsoreos, PhD, a neuroscientist at Rockefeller University. The reason: Levels of oxytocin (known as the "love hormone" to some) are sky-high upon waking, explains Karatsoreos, making it the best time for intimacy of all kinds.

Tap into It

These are the hours to strengthen your relationship with the most important people in your life. And if you wake up feeling frisky and need more than just cuddling, there's good news. Your husband's brain is on nearly the same wavelength; British researchers found high morning oxytocin levels in men—whether they were age 25 or 70—that gradually decreased as the day wore on. Now's a great time to:

- Make love or cuddle.
- Remind your partner how much you love him or her.
- Call your child at college (as long as it's not the weekend!).
- Write a thank-you note to a friend or relative.

9 TO 11 A.M.

Prime time for: Creativity

Your brain now has moderate levels of the stress hormone cortisol, which in reasonable amounts can actually help your mind focus, says Sung Lee, MD, secretary of the International Brain Education Association. It's present at any age: A University of Michigan study found that college students and retired adults were mentally quick in the morning, but among older subjects, sharpness declined in the afternoon.

Tap into It

Take on tasks that require analysis and concentration. "From middle age on, you're more alert early in the day," says Carolyn Yoon, PhD, an associate professor of marketing at the University of Michigan who worked on the study. Schedule discussions that involve personal or family matters, because others will be sharp at this time as well. Now's a great time to:

- Develop a new idea.
- Write a presentation.
- Brainstorm solutions to challenges large or small.
- Have an important conversation with your doctor.

11 A.M. TO 2 P.M.

Prime time for: Tough tasks

By now, levels of the sleep hormone melatonin have dipped sharply from their late evening and early morning peaks. This means you're more ready to take on a load of projects, according to German researchers. They found that reaction time and the ability to accomplish several to-dos were strong in the middle of the day.

Tap into It

Tear through your to-dos. Because of your mental quickness, this time of day is best for doing. One warning: Cross items off your list one at a time, says René Marois, PhD, an associate professor of psychology and neuroscience at Vanderbilt University. Attempts to juggle tasks put additional demands on your brain, he says. Faster reaction time can also help you respond briskly to your spouse's retorts during a dispute. Now's a great time to:

- Tackle your errand list, voice mails, or e-mails.
- Give a presentation to a client or boss.
- Iron out a tough problem with your spouse.

2 TO 3 P.M.

Prime time for: A break

To digest your lunch, your body draws blood away from your brain to your stomach, says Dr. Lee. Aim to eat a lunch closer to 2 p.m., because the midday meal can make you wish there were a couch close by. Your body's circadian rhythm (the biological "clock" that regulates sleep and wakefulness) is also in a brief down phase during this time, according to a recent Harvard study.

FIND YOUR BEST HOUR TO EXERCISE

Your ideal time of day for working out "depends on if you're a morning lark or a night owl," says neuroscientist Ilia Karatsoreos, PhD. According to researchers, there are at least two distinct chronotypes, a term that describes your body's response to circadian rhythms and in large part determines your optimal exercise hour. Want to switch yours?

If you have never been a morning workout person but that has become the only time you can do it, convert with these tips from *Prevention*'s fitness director, Michele Stanten.

- **EXERCISE WITH A FRIEND.** You're less likely to hit the snooze button if it means standing up someone.
- **LAY OUT YOUR GYM ATTIRE THE NIGHT BEFORE.** Some people even sleep in their workout clothes!
- **STICK TO YOUR ROUTINE.** Keep a similar sleep and wake schedule on the weekends, to avoid slipping out of your routine come Monday morning.
- **PUT YOUR ALARM CLOCK ACROSS THE ROOM.** That way, you're forced to get out of bed to turn it off.
- **CANCEL YOUR NEWSPAPER DELIVERY.** You'll have to walk (briskly) to the store in the morning to pick it up, as one *Prevention* reader did.

Tap into It

Take this time for yourself: Steer clear of work-related material and peruse your favorite publications instead. If you're at work and need to fight off drowsiness, Dr. Lee suggests a quick walk around the block or drink of water. Both of these actions will get your blood moving away from your stomach and toward your head. "Water increases vascular volume and circulation, promoting blood flow to your brain," he says. Now's a great time to:

- Meditate or pray.
- Read a magazine, the newspaper, or Web sites.
- Go for a brisk stroll.

3 TO 6 P.M.

Prime time for: Collaboration

"The brain is pretty fatigued by now," says Paul Nussbaum, PhD, an adjunct associate professor of neurological surgery at the University of Pittsburgh School of Medicine and author of *Your Brain Health Lifestyle*. That doesn't mean you're stressed, however: University of Michigan scientists found that cortisol levels usually decline in women by late afternoon.

Tap into It

Although you're not as mentally sharp as earlier, you're more easygoing, so plan a low-pressure meeting for now. If you've already left work, pick an activity that is as different from your job as possible, suggests Nussbaum. Exercise is a perfect one: Studies show that grip strength, manual dexterity, and other physical skills are at their strongest by the evening, but if you work out too late, the residual adrenaline can interfere with sleep. A gym session right before dinner solves the problem. Now's a great time to:

- Brainstorm with coworkers.
- Strength-train.

6 TO 8 P.M.

Prime time for: Personal tasks

Between these hours, researchers have found that the mind enters something called "wake maintenance," when its production of sleep-friendly melatonin is at an all-day low. As a result, chances of getting tired now are next to none. Studies also show that your taste buds are lit up during these hours because of circadian variations in hormone levels.

Tap into It

Keep your energy up by exposing yourself to the last of the day's serotonin-stimulating sunlight. Now may be a good time to walk the dog or walk to the corner store. And because you're now more alert but no longer at work, direct your renewed burst of mental energy toward your spouse and kids, and maybe some friends; you're bound to be pretty engaging about now. Now's a great time to:

- Run errands.
- Clean a long-overdue room in your house.
- Enjoy quality time with your family members.
- Make a delicious meal.

8 TO 10 P.M.

Prime time for: Relaxation

There's an abrupt transition from being wide awake to feeling sleepy as melatonin levels rise quickly, report Australian and British researchers. Meanwhile, levels of serotonin, a neurotransmitter tied to perkiness, start to fade: "Eighty percent of serotonin is stimulated from exposure to daylight, so now you're slowing down," says Rubin Naiman, PhD, an assistant professor of medicine at the University of Arizona and sleep program director at Miraval Resort in Tucson.

Tap into It

Now's the time to ease into relaxing, "mindless" activities (save the Sudoku for the morning). "By nightfall, when your brain is tired, this is a

HEALTH HEROES

She connects women who have the same kinds of breast cancer

When Vicki Tashman, 49, of Los Angeles, was diagnosed with invasive breast cancer, she researched the disease, found the best doctors, and took up meditation. Still, she felt frustrated and alone. So in 2006, she founded Pink-Link.org, the first Web site to connect breast cancer patients with others who share their exact diagnoses. "People don't realize how many different kinds of breast cancers there are and how treatment can vary," she says. "You want to talk to somebody who's been there."

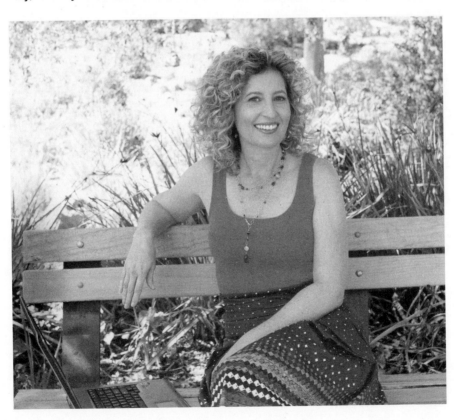

good way to bring yourself down, like walking a lap or two after a big workout," says Naiman. Now's a great time to:

Unwind by watching a funny movie.

Try a low-key, repetitive activity, such as taking a leisurely stroll or knitting.

10 P.M. ONWARD

Prime time to: Hit the sack

Your brain is looking to knit together all it learned today, which it does during sleep. Your top priority should be getting a full night's rest. Sleep can inspire insight: In a recent study, more than half of those taught a task thought of an easier way to do it after 8 hours of sleep. Adjusting lighting can help: Dim the rooms you occupy after dinner to let your body know the day is ending, suggests Naiman. In a few hours, your brain will be ready to start all over again.

Tap into It

Whatever helps you get to sleep—and it may take adjustments over time—follow your routine consistently. Just make sure you sign off early enough so you get the National Sleep Foundation's recommended 7 to 9 hours of shut-eye. Now's a great time to:

- Curl up with a good book.
- Write in your journal.
- Drift off while reading something you want to remember in the morning.

HAVE A GREAT DAY

Start every day off right with our three-step plan

Here's a wake-up call: What you do in the hour after you get up can help you look and feel your best for the rest of the day. The right moves and foods will give you the focus, stamina, and positive outlook you need to plow through your busy schedule. Plus, you'll kick-start your metabolism, helping you torch extra calories and melt more fat. Our get-up-and-go routine outlines the latest research-based tips guaranteed to make your morning a true power hour.

STEP 1: WAKE UP REFRESHED!

Even early birds can find it difficult to slip out from under their warm, cozy covers on dark winter mornings. Here's how to make it easier.

Note good things to come. Before going to bed, put a sticky note on your alarm clock reminding you of something fun or exciting that's happening the next day. "Because of hormonal shifts that occur while we're asleep, the majority of us wake up feeling a bit down or in a so-so mood," says Dana Lightman, PhD, a behavioral psychologist in Abington, Pennsylvania. "Remembering that you're having lunch with a friend or that your favorite TV show will be on that night gives you a quick lift."

Keep a cool bedroom. A toasty room temperature makes it easier to nod off, but you may wake up groggy. Lowering your thermostat right before turning out the lights maintains the warmth you need to fall asleep and will cool the room overnight—allowing you to rise and shine. Don't make it too chilly, though: Experts say the ideal temperature is between 60° and 70°F.

Surround yourself with color. "Seeing a bright, vibrant hue when you open your eyes gets your adrenaline going. That sudden surge of energy helps clear the cobwebs and kicks you into gear," says Leatrice Eiseman, executive director of the Pantone Color Institute. Put a red, orange, yellow, or fuchsia throw pillow, blanket, or piece of art in the area you first see in the morning, or slip on a robe in one of these shades. You can even make breakfast visually stimulating (and get a nutritional boost) by pouring yourself a glass of antioxidant-rich pomegranate or cranberry juice with a sweet slice of orange.

Put flowers by your bedside. Seeing a bouquet of blooms when they first woke up gave women in a new study a mood lift and energy boost that lasted all day, reports Nancy Etcoff, PhD, a faculty member at Harvard Medical School and the Harvard University Mind/Brain/Behavior Initiative.

Don't hit the snooze button. There's truth in the adage "You snooze, you lose." When you hit snooze, your brain knows it will go off again in a few minutes—so you won't go into the deeper, more restful stages of slumber. That means you'll be more tired than if you'd gotten up when it first sounded. A better strategy: "Set your alarm for when you really need to get up," says Jodi Mindell, PhD, associate director of the Sleep Disorders

Center at the Children's Hospital of Philadelphia. "That extra, uninterrupted sleep makes you feel more rested and refreshed when you get out of bed."

Visualize your day. Once you're awake, close your eyes and picture yourself alert and energetic. "Imagining an activity fires up the same parts of your brain that are used when you actually experience it," says Lightman. "Thinking positively about the day ahead energizes you."

Drink a big glass of water. This is a good way to replenish the fluid your body loses overnight, and it provides instant energy. "Everything that happens in your body requires water," says Holly Andersen, MD, an assistant professor of medicine at Weill Cornell Medical Center. "Without enough of it, your systems have to work harder in every respect—which can cause fatigue." Indeed, even a 2 percent drop in water stores can tire you physically and mentally. Starting to sip early also gives you a head start on the 11 cups of water the Institute of Medicine now recommends women consume throughout the day to stay hydrated.

Let the light in. A splash of sunlight makes you feel more awake, so read the paper by a sunny window or step outside for a few minutes while having your coffee. "Daylight signals your biological clock to stop the secretion of melatonin, a hormone that makes you sleepy, and promotes wakefulness," says James B. Maas, PhD, a professor and past chairman of the department of psychology at Cornell University. It also increases the brain's level of serotonin, which is a chemical that boosts mood.

If it's still dark when you get up, consider purchasing a dawn stimulator (from $80; lighttherapyproducts.com), a device that gradually brightens a light source at a preprogrammed time. Set it to create a dawn that breaks a half-hour before your usual wake-up time and grows to maximum brightness when your alarm goes off. Even when your eyes are closed, the light that passes through your lids signals your internal clock to trigger waking neurons in your brain.

Rub yourself awake. "Massaging your face boosts circulation, making it a surefire way to wake up," says Maggy Dunphy, general manager of the Aria Spa and Club in Vail, Colorado. Starting at your forehead and working down to your chin, lightly flutter-tap or drum your fingertips, varying the velocity, intensity, and location until you've touched your entire face. Bonus: Applying these moves will give you a quick healthy glow.

Have sex. Physical activity is one of the best ways to shake off grogginess. Plus having sex boosts your body's levels of chemicals associated with stamina (testosterone), energy (dopamine), and calmness (oxytocin), says Helen E. Fisher, PhD, a research professor in the department of anthropology at Rutgers University. What a great way to start the day!

STEP 2: GET ALL-DAY ENERGY

Nothing gives you a natural energy boost like exercise, which pumps fatigue-fighting oxygen to your cells and releases mood-boosting endorphins. Even a short session does the trick: In one study, workouts as brief as 10 minutes sparked energy levels for up to 2 hours. The 20-minute interval program below—which alternates brief bursts of high-intensity exercise with longer, slower segments—is ideal for a.m. exercisers.

"The intervals are invigorating and will get your heart rate up much quicker than walking at a slower, steady pace," says Tracey Mallett, a certified personal trainer in Los Angeles, who designed the workout. Another plus: Walking at a brisk pace burns more calories. Now that's something worth getting out of bed for!

Your Workout at a Glance

Do the Walking Program, followed by the Start-the-Day Stretches three to five times a week for a month, then increase the high-intensity intervals to 1 minute. (This will add an extra 2½ minutes to the workout.) To make the program harder and boost your fitness, increase the high-intensity intervals to 1½ minutes.

WALKING PROGRAM

TIME	PACE*
0:00–5:00 min	Warm up at a slow, even pace, working up to a light, leisurely stroll (an RPE of 4 to 5).
5:01–8:00 min	Quicken your pace slightly to an RPE of 6 (You should be able to converse.)
8:01–8:30 min	Walk as fast as you can. This pace should be challenging—an RPE of 7 to 8 (You'll find it harder to speak.)
8:31–10:30 min	Decrease to an easy pace—an RPE of 5 to 6.
10:31–11:00 min	Walk as fast as you can—an RPE of 7 to 8.
11:01–13:00 min	Decrease to an easy pace—an RPE of 5 to 6.
13:01–13:30 min	Walk as fast as you can—an RPE of 7 to 8.
13:31–15:30 min	Decrease to an easy pace—an RPE of 5 to 6.
15:31–16:00 min	Walk as fast as you can—an RPE of 7 to 8.
16:01–18:00 min	Decrease to an easy pace—an RPE of 5 to 6.
18:01–18:30 min	Walk as fast as you can—an RPE of 7 to 8.
18:31–20:30 min	Cool down; decrease to an easier pace, similar to the warmup.

*Pace yourself: Use the Rate of Perceived Exhaustion (RPE) to gauge how hard you feel you're working on a scale from 1 to 10, with 10 being the hardest.

Start-the-Day Stretches

Make time after your workout for these five standing stretches, which help keep your circulation revved, increasing your energy boost. As a bonus, most of the moves target the hardest working muscles in your body, including your thighs, hamstrings, and calves, which tend to be tightest in the a.m.

OVERHEAD REACH

TARGETS SHOULDERS AND CHEST

Stand tall, holding a rolled-up towel in front of you at shoulder height with hands shoulder-width apart. Keeping arms slightly bent, exhale and lift them up and overhead until you feel a gentle pull in chest and shoulders. Hold for 2 to 3 seconds, then return to starting position. Do 5 reps.

HIP OPENER

TARGETS HIP FLEXORS AND HAMSTRINGS

Stand with right foot about 2 feet in front of left foot. Bend right knee, bring hands down to floor on either side of right foot, and slide left foot back so leg is extended, left heel off floor. Hips should be level, right thigh parallel to floor, and right knee directly over right ankle. Hold for 30 seconds. Lower back knee to floor and shift hips back, extending right leg and raising right toes off floor. Hold for 30 seconds. Switch legs and repeat both parts of stretch.

FIGURE-FOUR STRETCH

TARGETS HIPS, GLUTES, AND INNER THIGHS

Holding on to a chair or wall, cross right leg on top of left thigh (just above knee). Bend left leg and press hips back as if you were going to sit down. Hold for 30 seconds; repeat with opposite leg.

CALF RELEASE

TARGETS CALVES

Holding on to a chair or wall, stand tall with right foot 1 to 2 feet in front of left, feet flat on floor and toes pointing forward. Bend right knee slightly until you feel a stretch in left calf. Don't roll onto the inside of feet. Hold for 30 seconds; switch legs and repeat. To increase the stretch, lean body slightly forward in a diagonal line from crown of head to heel.

STORK POSE

TARGETS THIGHS

Holding on to a chair or wall, bend right leg behind you and grasp right foot with right hand. Pull heel toward butt. Keep hips facing forward, abs pulled in, and pelvis still. Hold for 30 seconds; repeat with opposite leg.

STEP 3: BOOST YOUR FAT BURN

You'll reap benefits all day from eating breakfast: A morning meal shifts your body from an energy-conserving state into calorie-burning gear without effort. And studies show that breakfast eaters concentrate better and are more productive—as well as less likely to be obese—than breakfast skippers. These easy, satisfying recipes feature ingredients such as green tea that give your metabolism an added jolt.

BLUEBERRY AND GREEN TEA SMOOTHIE

2 SERVINGS ■ 334 CALORIES

Antioxidants abound in this refreshing—and filling—breakfast drink. Green tea and blueberries protect your cells from free radicals, which damage DNA in the mitochondria, the key players in your body's calorie-burning engine. Almonds provide natural protein and healthy monounsaturated fat, while flaxseed adds inflammation-fighting omega-3 fats to the mix. Brewing the tea the night before saves time in the morning. Drink one smoothie today and refrigerate the other serving for tomorrow.

¾ cup water

2 green tea bags

2 cups fresh or frozen blueberries

3 ice cubes

1½ cups fat-free vanilla yogurt

2 tablespoons whole dry-roasted, unsalted almonds (about 20)

2 tablespoons ground flaxseed

1. BRING the water to a boil and pour over the tea bags. Steep for 4 minutes. Squeeze and remove the tea bags and discard. Chill the tea overnight. If using fresh blueberries, place them in the freezer overnight.

2. PLACE the tea, blueberries, ice, yogurt, almonds, and flaxseed in a blender. Process until smooth.

NUTRITION PER SERVING

334 calories, 13 g protein, 55 g carbohydrates, 8.5 g fat, 1 g saturated fat, 3 mg cholesterol, 121 mg sodium, 7 g fiber

CRANBERRY-ORANGE OAT PANCAKES

8 SERVINGS ■ **259 CALORIES**

Prepare these ahead of time, freeze them, and reheat for the convenience of the boxed variety without the empty calories of refined carbs. Fiber-rich oats and whole wheat flour keep your metabolism in high gear and your cravings in check.

1 cup old-fashioned rolled oats

1 cup whole wheat flour

¼ cup all-purpose flour

3 tablespoons packed brown sugar

4 teaspoons baking powder

1 teaspoon ground cinnamon

¼ teaspoon salt

2 large eggs

1 cup orange juice

¼ cup 2% milk

¼ cup extra virgin olive oil or canola oil

¾ cup sweetened dried cranberries

Agave nectar, for serving

1. PREHEAT a nonstick griddle (if using electric griddle, set to 325° to 350°F).

2. WHISK together the oats, whole wheat flour, all-purpose flour, sugar, baking powder, cinnamon, and salt in a large bowl. In a medium bowl, whisk together the eggs, orange juice, milk, and oil.

3. ADD the wet ingredients to the dry ingredients and stir to combine. Fold in the cranberries.

4. DROP ¼ cup of the batter onto the griddle and cook until the edges look dry and bubbles come to the surface, about 3 minutes. Flip and cook until the bottom browns and the pancake is cooked through, 1 to 2 minutes. Repeat with remaining the batter. Serve with the agave nectar.

NUTRITION PER SERVING

259 calories, 6 g protein, 39 g carbohydrates, 9.5 g fat, 1.5 g saturated fat, 53 mg cholesterol, 298 mg sodium, 4 g fiber

KITCHEN CURE

You don't have to drink coffee to experience its eye-opening effects. An international group of scientists found that just smelling coffee helped drowsy rats feel better. The aroma boosted antioxidant activity in the brain. If you're fighting that afternoon droop, try a sniff instead of a sip of coffee.

EGG, CHEESE, AND BACON SANDWICH

1 SERVING ■ 279 CALORIES

Our protein- and fiber-packed breakfast sandwich satisfies a hearty appetite with only 10 percent of the cholesterol and about half of the sodium of the healthiest similar drive-thru choice. Spinach is what sets it apart: The leafy green provides vitamins A and K and iron, plus coenzyme Q10, which is a compound required for a well-tuned metabolism. No time to cook in the morning? Make a sandwich the night before and reheat it in the microwave the next day.

1 slice (1 ounce) lower-sodium bacon

½ teaspoon extra virgin olive oil

¼ cup liquid egg substitute

1 light multigrain English muffin, toasted

1½ ounces trimmed spinach leaves or baby spinach (about 1 cup packed)

Freshly ground black pepper

¾ ounce slice reduced-fat, reduced-sodium Swiss or Jarlsberg cheese

1. MICROWAVE the bacon slice per package directions.

2. HEAT the oil in a small nonstick skillet over medium heat. Add the egg substitute and heat until the edges begin to set, about 1 minute. Lift the edges to allow any liquid egg to flow underneath, and cook about 1 minute longer. When almost set, gently fold the omelet in half and in half again. Transfer to the bottom half of the muffin and top with the bacon.

3. RETURN the pan to the heat, add the spinach, and cook, stirring until wilted, about 1 minute. Place the spinach on top of the bacon, season with the pepper, add the cheese, and top with the other muffin half.

NUTRITION PER SANDWICH

279 calories, 23 g protein, 27 g carbohydrates, 12.5 g fat, 5 g saturated fat, 26 mg cholesterol, 428 mg sodium, 9 g fiber

MAGNIFY YOUR BRAINPOWER

Focus your concentration with these tips—and discover how smart you really are

Christine Grote was driving to a shopping mall 18 miles from her home in Cincinnati when she realized that she had been traveling in the wrong direction for nearly 20 minutes. "I was thinking about a job interview and lost track of where I was headed," says the 51-year-old mother of four. "I didn't get in an accident, but my mind certainly wasn't on driving—it was frightening."

Scary, yes, but also predictable, experts say: Your brain is naturally primed to wander whenever it can, according to a joint study by Harvard University, Dartmouth College, and the University of Aberdeen in Scotland. Using MRI, researchers found that brain regions responsible for task-unrelated thought (that is, daydreaming or mind wandering) are almost constantly active when the brain is at rest or performing a task that doesn't require concentration.

Fortunately, brain experts say it's possible to corral that brainpower, filter out distractions, and master any task by improving your concentration. Here are their top tips for refocusing.

CAN'T CONCENTRATE AT WORK?

Unless you love everything about your job, you're bound to zone out occasionally, according to a study at the University of North Carolina at Greensboro. Among 124 people, mind wandering occurred about 30 percent of the time, even during crucial tasks—adding up to many hours of lost productivity. Boredom, fatigue, and stress all spur mind wandering, says study author Michael Kane, PhD, an associate professor of psychology at UNC. And although women were no more likely than men to lose focus, they reported general worrying and anxiety when their attention drifted. Fear not: Some mind wandering is simply your brain taking a healthy break, although sometimes it's best left for another occasion.

Organize to eliminate distractions. If you have several to-dos, decide which to tackle first and clear all other projects off your desk and

KITCHEN CURE

To keep your mind sharp, snack on celery and green bell peppers. Luteolin, a plant compound abundant in these two green vegetables, can prevent inflammation in the brain linked with aging and diseases such as Alzheimer's and multiple sclerosis, according to researchers at the University of Illinois. The scientists studied the compound's effect on human brain cells in a test tube and on mice, and in both cases found that it decreased inflammation.

Try dipping celery and green bell pepper slices in hummus, or chop and mix with tuna, herbs (such as parsley or chives), and a dollop of plain yogurt for a healthy tuna salad.

computer screen. "Out of sight, out of mind applies," Kane says. "Get rid of memos, e-mails, and anything else that reminds you you're behind."

Go easy on your cubicle's decor. You could be your own worst enemy. "Even family photos are potential thought stealers. They're people you're prone to worry about," Kane adds.

Participate. If you daydream during meetings, challenge yourself by thinking of questions for the speaker and raising your hand as much as possible, suggests Jonathan W. Schooler, PhD, a professor of psychology at the University of California, Santa Barbara. You may miss a moment when you're formulating your question, but it will help you stay focused on the current topic.

Relocate. When you start to lose concentration, leave your desk and take a walk outside or to the office common space for a mental breather. This way, your brain associates your desk only with work, not mind wandering. Warns Schooler: "If you don't take regular breaks—especially when you're not enjoying your job—your brain will take them for you."

DRIVING THE CAR ON AUTOPILOT?

We're most likely to space out during activities we can do automatically, according to a 2006 study. This is dangerous when you're behind the wheel: If a car ahead stops suddenly, your reaction time may not be fast enough to prevent an accident.

Tie a string around your steering wheel. When you think about the same things during your commute—anticipating the day's workload or what to cook for dinner—your brain begins to associate the car with zoning out, says Kane. A novel, visual cue such as a colored string or a dashboard sticker can snap you out of your "dream driving" habit.

Play a car game. Those involving counting or geography are great ways for kids to pass the time en route—for good reason: The contests use things that you should be aware of while driving. Try tallying all the states represented by the license plates of the cars in front of you.

(continued on page 248)

POTS OF HEALTH

Interior decorators know that a potted plant can add life to a room, but these leafy greens are more than just pretty accent pieces—they can reduce stress, zap environmental toxins, and even help you think more clearly. We dug through decades of research to find the feel-good effects of mixing a few houseplants into your home decor, from boosting your creativity to beating the sniffles. Experts say you should amass as much green as possible. (Your body will thank you, and so will your wallet—have you ever compared the cost of a fern with the price of a Picasso?)

Here are the best plants for every room—and exactly what to do to reap their health benefits. Blooms away!

To Destress

Put a dragon tree in the room with the smallest windows.

A little green can instantly chill you out, finds a recent survey from Sweden. City dwellers there who frequently visited areas with grass and trees reported fewer feelings of burnout and panic than those who rarely saw greenery. It's not entirely clear why, but many studies have found something similar, says Virginia I. Lohr, PhD, a professor at Washington State University who has been studying the subject for more than 30 years. It's suggested that evolution wired humans to know that plants are essential to survival, so seeing one makes us calm and settled.

In one of Lohr's studies, people who worked in a windowless computer lab that had common houseplants such as bamboo palm, Chinese evergreen, snake plant, or arrowhead vine (all can grow well in low-light settings) had a 4-point drop in their systolic blood pressure after taking a stressful computer-based test, compared with only a 2-point drop in a group that had no exposure to plants. That extra 2 points is equivalent to taking about half a blood pressure pill, and "every point counts," says Douglas Reifler, MD, a professor of general internal medicine at Northwestern University.

To Spark Creativity

Decorate your office with small but colorful African violets.

In a study from Texas A&M University, women who worked for an hour in a room decorated with two potted plants and a bouquet of flowers generated 13 percent more ideas than women in a room with abstract sculptures. Studies show that plants are a mood booster, and good moods are associated with higher levels of dopamine, the hormone that controls the flow of information throughout the brain. Your next bright idea: Head to a nursery or garden store and pick up a few houseplants of your own.

To Fight Colds

Place an ultra-leafy plant, such as a philodendron, in your bedroom.

Dry air can lead to a parched nose and throat—and raise the risk of infection or run-of-the-mill sinusitis, says Michael Janson, MD, author of *User's Guide to Heart-Healthy Supplements*. But houseplants can inject moisture back into the air and boost humidity by up to 5 percent, finds research from Bavarian State Institute of Viticulture and Horticulture in Germany. A humidifier would do more, but the natural boost from plants is enough to help alleviate symptoms. According to a study from the Agricultural University of Norway, people with table and floor-standing plants in their offices reported 37 percent less coughing and 25 percent less hoarseness after 3 months than when they left their offices plant free.

The researchers used heart-leaf philodendron among other plants, but you can choose the greens that are most appealing to you. Just pick a plant that has a lot of leaves, because these types release the most moisture, says Sarada Krishnan, director of horticulture at the Denver Botanic Gardens. To fight dry air while you sleep, try any indoor ivy variety, such as English ivy, or peace lilies and African violets. The more plants you have, the greater the benefit. Grab a few large pots and plant several smaller varieties in each.

(continued)

POTS OF HEALTH (*cont.*)

To Cut Exposure to Harmful Chemicals

All plants filter toxins from the air—so pick your favorite and put it next to your printer.

If you use a lot of cleaning supplies, or if you have a printer or newly painted walls or varnished furniture, you have VOCs (volatile organic compounds)—toxins that can cause dizziness, fatigue, nausea, kidney or liver damage, and even cancer. A study from the University of Technology in Sydney, Australia, looked at the ability of two widely available houseplants—the Janet Craig (a standing plant) and the Sweet Chico (a smaller table plant)—to strip VOCs from the air. Researchers found that five Sweet Chicos and one Janet Craig may reduce VOCs in a 130-square-foot room (such as a guest bedroom) by up to 70 percent.

When plants take in oxygen and carbon dioxide, they also pull in any toxins floating around in the air, says Kyle Wallick, a botanist at the United States Botanic Garden in Washington, DC. The toxins travel through the plant, ending up near the roots. There, bacteria in the soil break down the chemicals into nontoxic compounds that the plant uses for food.

For more healthy plant ideas, be sure to check out our slide show at Prevention.com/houseplants.

READING THE SAME PASSAGES IN A BOOK?

Don't blame a poor memory. "Mindless reading" is common and requires considerable effort to control, says Schooler, who found that readers are actually mind wandering about 20 percent of the time: "Their eyes move across the page, but they're not thinking about the text," he says.

Read actively. Take time-outs to process the material; mentally recap plot points or a character's motive, for example. "Periodically think over what you've read. It can improve comprehension, probably because it reduces mind wandering," Schooler says.

Read backward for a bit. If you glossed over a few paragraphs, read them in reverse—reordering small packets of information can sometimes change how much of it you absorb. It may feel odd at first, but the extra effort required will force your brain back into focusing.

Give up on dull books. As you might expect, studies show that you're most likely to drift when you're not interested in the material that you are trying to read. If a book doesn't grab you after a chapter or two, choose a new one.

Join a book club. A little peer pressure to finish a book by a certain date can go a long way, especially if you're expected to talk about the content. Budget the number of pages you'll need to read daily, and if you own the book, write notes in the margin and mark meaningful passages to boost both concentration and comprehension.

PREOCCUPIED BY A PERSONAL ISSUE?

People who report being unhappy, usually because of a difficult problem, have more intense mind wandering during tasks than their carefree counterparts, according to studies by Jonathan Smallwood, PhD, a lecturer at the University of Aberdeen's school of psychology. These feelings

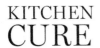

KITCHEN CURE

Researchers at MIT discovered that it may be possible to get smarter by eating smarter. They fed gerbils a diet enriched with compounds that the brain needs to maintain healthy membranes: choline (found in eggs); uridine monophosphate, or UMP (found in beets); and docosahexaenoic acid, or DHA (found in fish oils). After 4 weeks, the gerbils given the enriched diet performed better in various gerbil activities, such as mazes, than the gerbils that were fed standard food. The brains of the higher-functioning rodents had more synapse activity, which typically indicates a higher intelligence.

MEDITATE FOR GREATER MINDFULNESS

Meditation, a proven stress reliever, may also let you tune out distractions. Amishi Jha, PhD, an assistant professor of psychology at the University of Pennsylvania, studied attention control in people before and after they learned mindfulness meditation (sitting quietly for 30 minutes a day, focusing on breathing; when the subjects noticed their mind drifting, they gently guided their thoughts back to their breath). After 8 weeks they showed significant improvements at "orienting," or staying on task and quickly refocusing their thinking after being distracted. "Meditation trains you to put your attention where you want it and make sure it stays there," Jha says. To learn other meditation techniques, visit Prevention.com/meditate.

limit your ability to focus on anything else, he says: "You may spend a lot of time thinking about a problem when you're upset, but this type of ruminating is actually quite unproductive."

Get it off your chest. Talk about your worries with a friend or family member, either in person or on the telephone, to clear your head. Writing down your thoughts may be as effective as saying them out loud: List ways to address the problem and then move on, recommends Eric Klinger, PhD, a professor emeritus of psychology at the University of Minnesota, Morris, who has studied thought patterns during daydreams. "Committing a plan to paper helps put the problem on the back burner, so you can shift your attention to other things," he explains.

fast fact ---
90: The percentage of electronics in the United States that are not recycled
----

HEALTH HEROES

She protects people from hazardous waste

Labeled developmentally delayed as a kid, Lorraine Kerwood never thought she'd use a computer. Now, it's the 47-year-old's passion. In 2002, she founded Oregon-based Next-Step Recycling, which has refurbished 15,000 computers for disadvantaged communities and recycled 6 million pounds of other electronics—keeping them out of dumps, where their toxic parts are likely to pollute air and water supplies. "I have seven grandkids. I want to preserve our environment for them," she says.

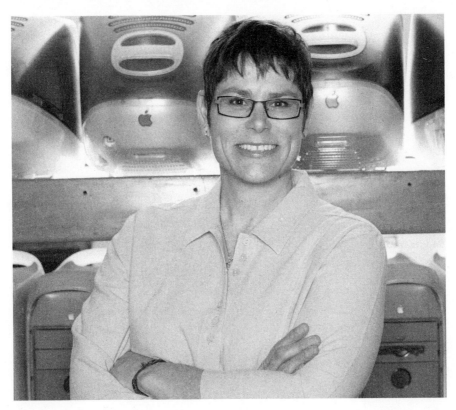

BE HAPPY

Scientists know that positive people are happier, period. Tapping into your bright side is easier than you'd guess

Joie de vivre. We all know people whose engagement with life can only be described as joyful (They're the ones who don't seem to get steamed when they're trapped in the slow-moving supermarket line, cut off by the land yacht on the freeway, or put on hold for 23 minutes by customer service.) Fittingly, nature rewards these happy-go-lucky types: Being optimistic in middle age increases life span by at least 7.5 years—even after accounting for age, gender, socioeconomic status, and physical health, according to a large Yale University survey. What's behind their hardiness: They minimize the destructive effects of stress.

"Of course, optimists get stressed," says David Snowdon, a professor of neurology at the University of Kentucky who studies aging. "But they automatically turn the response off much more quickly and return to a positive mental and physical state." Here are four habits that longevity experts say are at the heart of people with a sunny disposition—and that you can adopt, too.

THE BEST KIND OF PESSIMIST

If you're an irritable sort who thinks of your eternally cheery neighbor as a delusional Pollyanna, are you doomed to poor health? Not if you're an active pessimist, a feisty spirit who loves to complain, criticize, and generally mix it up with others—but then takes action.

"Active pessimists do battle with life. Being that engaged is actually good for them and can provide some of the same benefits that optimists enjoy," says Toni Antonucci, PhD, director of the Life Course Development Program of the Institute for Social Research at the University of Michigan. Passive pessimists, on the other hand, feel paralyzed by gloom, have given up on themselves and life, and will likely live fewer years because of their bummer attitude.

THEY WORK THEIR CELL PHONES

Perhaps your neighborhood gossip is on to something: All that chitchat keeps her plugged into a thriving social network, and people who socialize at least once a week are more likely to live longer, keep their brains sharp, and prevent heart attacks. One reason: "Just talking on the phone to a friend has the immediate effect of lowering your blood pressure and cortisol levels," says Teresa Seeman, PhD, a professor of medicine and epidemiology at UCLA. "Our research shows that having good long-term relationships provides as many physical benefits as being active or a nonsmoker."

Make the effort to connect with the friends you already have. Call now, and before you hang up, schedule a lunch date. Personal contact is even better.

THEY EXPRESS GRATITUDE (WITHIN REASON)

Buoy your spirits by recording happy events on paper, your computer, or a PDA. People who write about all the things they are thankful for are optimistic about the upcoming week and more satisfied overall with their lives, according to a University of California, Davis, study. They also feel physically stronger.

"It's hard to be bitter and mad when you're feeling grateful," says Sonja Lyubomirsky, PhD, author of the upcoming book *The How of Happiness: A Scientific Approach to Getting the Life You Want.*

But don't overdo it. Women who kept a gratitude journal only once a week got a bigger boost in happiness than those asked to record their good fortune three times a week. Find the frequency that works for you— giving thanks shouldn't feel like a chore.

THEY'RE RANDOMLY KIND

Do you perform five acts of kindness in any given day? That's the number of good deeds that boosts your sense of well-being and happiness, according to research by Lyubomirsky. Your karmic acts can be minor and unplanned—giving up your seat on the bus; buying an extra latte to give to a coworker. You'll find that the payback greatly exceeds the effort. "You see how much you're appreciated and liked by others," she says.

Be sure to keep up the good work: When Lyubomirsky asked her study subjects to space their five good deeds over the course of a week, the actions started to seem routine and lost some of their therapeutic effects. But don't fret if you can't make the quota daily. "Being spontaneously kind also delivers rewards," she says.

THEY REAPPRAISE THEIR LIVES

Yes, you can rewrite history—and feel better about yourself in the bargain. Set aside a little time each week to write about or record—or even just mentally revisit—an important event in your past. Reflecting on the experience can reshape your perception of it, as well as your expectations

THE GOOD MOOD DIET

Certain snacks make potent antidepressants, if you eat them right. Perhaps as a child whenever you visited your grandfather, you shared all sorts of cookies, always paired with a large glass of cold milk. Over the years they became so closely associated with visiting Granddad that now, whenever you have one, you feel buoyed by a swell of happy memories.

As it turns out, scientists have a solid explanation for that burst of good cheer, explains Thomas Crook, PhD, a clinical psychologist who has conducted extensive research to improve our understanding of how the brain works. Studies by Richard Wurtman, MD, and Judith Wurtman, PhD, at MIT have shown that snacking on readily digested carbohydrates, such as those in a cookie or bagel, can raise the brain's level of the chemical serotonin, the very same target of modern antidepressant medication.

Of course, other foods are reputed mood boosters, too—though their reputations may not always be deserved. Let's look at a few.

TEA: It's known as "the cup that cheers," and the caffeine in it can certainly improve energy. But that's a physiological response; no studies have confirmed a direct effect on your spirits. Mood booster? The jury's out. (The same is true of coffee.)

ALCOHOL: It's commonly thought of as a good-times libation, but it has a dark side. Although a recent study found that moderate drinkers (two drinks a day for men, one for women) had fewer depression symptoms than nondrinkers did, scores of other studies have established that alcohol in large quantities can be a devastating depressant. Mood booster? Perhaps, but only in small amounts.

for the future, says Robert N. Butler, MD, president of the International Longevity Center-USA in New York City. When creating this "life review," you get to list all your accomplishments—an instant self-esteem booster.

Organize your historical review by epochs: your postcollege years, early marriage, career, parenthood. Subdivide each section into triumphs, missteps, and lessons for the future. It's helpful to look at the bad times as well as the good. Perhaps now that a few years have passed, you'll be

CHOCOLATE: Many of us reach for it as a pick-me-up, but Australian scientists concluded that eating the sweet to lift your spirits "is more likely to prolong than abort the dysphoric [depressed] mood. It is not, as some would claim, an antidepressant." Mood booster? Apparently not. (Stick to a 1-ounce serving if you want to benefit from chocolate's disease-fighting antioxidants.)

GRANDDAD'S COOKIES: They can brighten your spirits when eaten judiciously. (Incidentally, carb snacking may be more effective for women because they produce substantially less serotonin than men do.) Now, you don't want to try this regimen if you have diabetes or are prediabetic. But if you qualify, try raising your mood-lifting serotonin levels a couple of times a day by doing the following.

INCLUDE PROTEIN IN EACH OF YOUR THREE MEALS. This will raise blood levels of tryptophan, which is a chemical that eventually turns into serotonin. The best sources of tryptophan are poultry, seafood, and lean meat.

HAVE A SMALL CARBOHYDRATE SNACK 3 or 4 hours after each meal and about 1 hour before your next one. Make sure that your stomach is empty and that you eat no protein between meals. The carbohydrates should be easily digestible—such as one or two oatmeal cookies, a third of a bagel, or a slice of whole wheat bread. This will cause tryptophan in your blood to enter the brain, where it is metabolized into serotonin. Elevated serotonin will improve your mood within 20 to 30 minutes.

If you follow the rules, you'll also fall asleep more quickly at night, because at the end of the day, your brain metabolizes serotonin into the natural sleep aid melatonin. From happy to sleepy, all by way of a cookie. It doesn't get much cheerier than that!

able to see how that breakup or failed job opportunity opened other doors and finally forgive yourself—and your ex-boyfriend or would-be boss.

"Even if a memory is painful, it's good to work through it," says Dr. Butler. "If you can come to terms with past events, you'll be better able to handle tough times down the road."

So be honest, but also go easy on yourself. Remember: You are the hero or heroine in this tale.

CHAPTER 30

THINK FAST

Misplaced your keys—again? Can't remember someone's name? These 8 breakthrough tips will help you fight forgetfulness

Is your memory in a state of rebellion? Most of us can certainly remember all the big things: our names, what year it is, our birth dates. But it's the little things—what you ate last week at that new restaurant or even whether you liked that new restaurant (speaking of which, what was its name?)—that sometimes slip away. Experts say that such "senior moments" are normal even if it will be decades before you can begin to think about tapping your 401(k). Reassuring, yes, but that still doesn't help you remember the name of that restaurant.

Brain researchers are on the case. Studies are uncovering how our mundane, everyday habits—what we eat, the pills we take, how we rest, and even our confidence levels—have a big impact on our brains. Here's what experts say are the newest strategies guaranteed to keep your memory quick, agile, and sharp.

CHECK YOUR IRON

Iron helps the neurotransmitters essential to memory function properly, and your brain can be sensitive to low amounts. "A poor diet or heavy menstrual periods, such as those during perimenopause, can cause your iron levels to drop enough to affect your recall abilities, even if you don't have anemia," says Laura Murray-Kolb, PhD, an assistant professor of international health at Johns Hopkins University. When she gave memory tests to 149 women, those with low iron levels missed twice as many questions as those with sufficient amounts. Yet after 4 months of taking iron supplements, most of the women, with their iron levels back to normal, scored as well as the best group in the first test. Murray-Kolb recom-

HIGH-TECH BRAIN POWER

What's an eight-letter word for brain booster? The answer could be Nintendo. Experts say playing one of the new games specially designed to improve your focus could have the indirect effect of getting your memory in shape.

"Whenever you solve puzzles or do brainteasers, you're making the connections between your neurons work more efficiently, which is like putting money in the bank," says Stuart Zola, PhD, an Alzheimer's researcher at Emory University. But if you get too good at one game, you should quickly proceed to the next level, or try a new one altogether. Your brain is very much like a muscle: It needs constant challenge to grow.

For starters, try the following.

- *Nintendo's Brain Age*, which is a computer game featuring a set of fun reading and mathematical exercises to be done every day.
- A "virtual mental gymnasium" at MyBrainTrainer.com, where you can calculate your "brain age" and work to lower it.
- Prevention.com/braingames for games from the "brain fitness" experts at Happy Neuron.

mends that women who don't get enough through their diets consider taking a daily multivitamin with 18 milligrams of iron (8 milligrams for postmenopausal women).

If you still suspect you're low, ask your doctor for a blood test to check your ferritin level, which will reveal even a moderate iron deficiency; a regular blood test isn't sensitive enough to pick up levels lower than the threshold for anemia.

TURN OFF BACKGROUND NOISE

We all multitask, a necessary survival skill of the digital age. But did you know that just listening to the news while you answer your e-mail can limit how well you're able to recall both? Normally, when you take in new information, you process it with a part of the brain called the cerebral cortex. "But multitasking greatly reduces learning because people can't attend to the relevant information," says UCLA psychology professor and memory researcher Russell Poldrack, PhD. That's because the brain is forced to switch processing to an area called the striatum, and the information stored there tends to contain fewer important details.

Luckily, this kind of memory problem has an easy fix, says Poldrack: Simply pay undivided attention to whatever you really want to recall.

REFRESH YOUR MIND

Yes, you know that meditation can reduce stress, which research shows can damage brain cells and your ability to retain information over time. But the ancient practice can do more than just soothe your soul: It may also sharpen your memory. According to a University of Kentucky study, subjects who took a late-afternoon test after meditating for 40 minutes had significantly better scores than those who napped for the same period. Even more surprising, when the subjects were retested after being deprived of a full night's sleep, those who meditated still scored better than their study counterparts.

How could that be? Meditation, like sleep, reduces sensory input, and this quiet state may provide a time for neurons to process and solidify new information and memories. Brain scans have revealed that meditation produces a state somewhat similar to non-REM sleep (which many specialists believe is the more mentally restorative sleep phase), in that many neurons of the cortex fire in sync, says Bruce O'Hara, PhD, a coauthor of the study. "However, unlike when you sleep, consciousness is fully maintained in meditation, so there is no grogginess upon 'awakening.'"

For regular, highly experienced meditators, the benefits to memory can be substantial. A University of Wisconsin–Madison study discovered that the brains of long-term Buddhist practitioners who have meditated every day for many years generated the highest levels of gamma waves—a pattern of brain activity that's associated with attention, working memory, and learning—ever reported in other studies.

Here are some good sources to help you get started.

A Woman's Book of Meditation: Discovering the Power of a Peaceful Mind by Hari Kaur Khalsa

Meditation for Beginners DVD (gaiam.com)

CONTROL YOUR CHOLESTEROL

A healthful cholesterol level is as essential for mental sharpness as it is for cardiovascular efficiency. When plaque, caused by "bad" LDL cholesterol, builds up in blood vessels, it can hinder circulation to the brain, depriving it of essential nutrients. One possible consequence: memory problems.

"It doesn't take much plaque to block the tiny blood vessels in the brain," explains Aaron P. Nelson, PhD, chief of psychology and neuropsychology at Brigham and Women's Hospital in Boston. "In addition, several studies have shown that high cholesterol is a risk factor for Alzheimer's disease." Although that connection is not fully understood, the take-home is clear: Get your cholesterol checked regularly; if it's high, work with your doctor to lower it.

DOUBLE-CHECK YOUR MEDS

One side effect of taking many prescription and over-the-counter drugs can be a worrisome increase in memory lapses. Antidepressants, anti-anxiety drugs, antispasmodics, beta-blockers, chemotherapy, Parkinson's medications, sleeping pills, ulcer medications, painkillers, antihistamines, and even statins can all affect your memory, says Gary Small, MD, chief of the UCLA Memory and Aging Research Center and author of *The Longevity Bible: 8 Essential Strategies for Keeping Your Mind Sharp and Your Body Young.*

As you get older, drugs tend to stay in your system for a longer period of time, increasing the likelihood of troublesome interactions. Fortunately, any drug-related impairment will likely improve as soon as the drug is discontinued. "Speaking with your doctor about adjusting your dose or switching medications is often a simple solution," says Dr. Small.

SNACK ON FRUIT

A couple of apples a day may actually keep the *neurologist* away. And so might blueberries. Both fruits appear to have some significant memory-boosting qualities.

KITCHEN CURE

Red wine may help preserve your memory. According to research done by Philippe Marambaud, PhD, a compound in red wine, resveratrol, may help ward off Alzheimer's disease.

Marambaud, a senior research scientist at New York's Litwin-Zucker Research Center for the Study of Alzheimer's Disease and Memory Disorders, found in lab experiments that resveratrol hampered the formation of beta-amyloid protein, which is a key ingredient in plaque found in the brains of people who die with Alzheimer's disease.

Alcohol's benefits to the heart (it can help lower cholesterol levels) may also protect against memory loss by improving circulation to the brain, says Aaron P. Nelson, PhD, chief of psychology and neuropsychology at Brigham and Women's Hospital in Boston. But remember, everything in moderation: "Drinking more than a glass won't help, and it just might hurt."

"Apples have just the right dose of antioxidants to raise levels of acetylcholine, a neurotransmitter that's essential to memory and tends to decline with age," says Tom Shea, PhD, director of the University of Massachusetts Lowell Center for Cellular Neurobiology and Neurodegeneration Research. In addition, antioxidants in apples help preserve memory by protecting brain cells against damage from free radicals created by everyday metabolic action, such as the processing of glucose by the body's cells.

A study by Shea and Amy Chan, PhD, found that mice suffering from the equivalent of normal human age-related memory loss or early Alzheimer's disease got a memory boost when they consumed a daily dose of apple juice. After just 1 month, those mice did a far superior job on a maze, which tests short-term memory, than the animals that didn't get the drink. Shea has begun clinical trials to determine whether humans get a similar benefit. For right now, he recommends consuming two or three apples or two 8-ounce glasses of apple juice each day; even one will give your brain a good lift.

Researchers have long touted blueberries as a rich source of flavonoids, particularly anthocyanins and flavanols, but it's never been clear how they affect the brain, until now. A study at the University of Reading and the Peninsula Medical School in England has provided some intriguing insight. The study suggests that when flavonoids are ingested, they cross the blood-brain barrier to help improve the functioning of brain cells. Flavonoids even appear to help regenerate new brain cells. The participants in the study ate a diet supplemented with 10 ounces of blueberries every day for 12 weeks. The results showed improvements of recall-test scores after just 3 weeks of eating the fruit. Those improvements continued throughout the study.

The research team plans to take these findings further and study the effects of flavonoids on Alzheimer's disease and other forms of cognitive impairment. In the meantime, grab a handful of these juicy beauties to give your brain a burst of antioxidants.

REV UP YOUR HEART

Old-fashioned cardio can also keep your memory spry by improving a number of brain functions. Researchers from the University of Illinois, Urbana, put two groups of older, healthy adult volunteers on different regimens. One group did aerobic training three times a week for 1 hour; the other did nonaerobic stretching and toning. MRIs taken after 3 months showed that the aerobics group actually increased their brains' volume (which could reflect new neurons or cells) and white matter (connections between neurons) in the frontal lobes, which contribute to attention and memory processing. The aerobic exercisers, who ranged from age 60 to 79, had the brain volumes of people 2 to 3 years younger, said Arthur Kramer, PhD, who reported his results in the *Journal of Gerontology: Medical Sciences*. Taking a 1-hour walk at a brisk, slightly breathless pace three times a week will likely confer the same benefits.

BELIEVE IN YOUR BRAIN

Do you find yourself worrying about forgetfulness? Give it up! Any anxiety you feel about your occasionally wayward memory later in life may actually make it worse. In a North Carolina State University study published in *Psychology and Aging*, healthy older adults scored poorly on memory tests after being informed that aging causes forgetfulness. When another group was told that there wasn't much of a decline in their recall abilities with age, however, they scored 15 percent higher—even better than a control group told nothing about memory and age.

"Believing in negative stereotypes can be a self-fulfilling prophecy," says head researcher and psychology professor Thomas M. Hess, PhD. "That's a shame, because your memory probably isn't nearly as bad as you fear it is."

BE A POWER PERSUADER

Get your spouse, friends—and anyone else—to do things your way with these research-tested tips

When toddlers don't get what they want, they jump up and down, howl at the top of their lungs, and throw things. No matter how tempting these options may be, they just aren't open to adults. We need more subtle ways to sway people to our sides.

Getting a great deal on a new car, talking your spouse into taking a vacation, enlisting reluctant coworkers to adopt your big idea, recruiting friends to a cause—all require clever powers of persuasion. Luckily, emerging research by psychologists, economists, and other experts can arm you with the skills you need to have things your way. Here's your cheat sheet.

GET YOUR SPOUSE TO AGREE

Be a problem solver. Women are more deft at resolving conflict than their husbands are, according to a new study by Iowa State University psychologists. That doesn't mean that women should use their skills to always get their way. Instead, rely on superior problem-solving abilities to take the lead in finding areas of compromise.

A good way to start: Give a minor dispute—for example, where to vacation—the attention it deserves and ask your spouse to do the same, advises Carnegie Mellon University economist Linda Babcock, PhD, coauthor of the new book *Ask for It: How Women Can Use the Power of Negotiation to Get What They Really Want.*

Your Strategy

Focus on similarities. Don't just say to your spouse, "I want to go to Key West." That's an intractable position, explains Babcock. Instead, talk about what you want out of your trip ("I'd like to go sailing and spend time at the beach"). Then suggest that your partner do the same, and seek common ground. You may find another seaside locale that features the activities that appeal to both of you, such as a location that has a PGA golf course *and* sun and sand. "Find a resolution in the places where your interests intersect," says Babcock.

INFLUENCE COWORKERS

State your case over and over. When one person expresses an opinion repeatedly—in a friendly way—the effect is the same as several people lobbying the point, a study found. Repetition evokes a sense of familiarity, making it seem that convictions are widely shared, says study coauthor Stephen Garcia, PhD, of the University of Michigan Gerald R. Ford School of Public Policy.

Your Strategy

Repeat your message in their words. Before pushing an idea at work, practice mimicking your coworkers' communication styles, suggests Caroline Keating, PhD, a psychology professor at Colgate University. If your coworker leans in slightly while talking to you, do the same, and mirror her speech pattern.

"Get in sync nonverbally with the other person. It's much easier to agree with someone if you're on the same wavelength," says Keating. As you're enjoying that easy rapport, refer to your idea a few times in a positive tone. To increase the likelihood that your idea is given priority at work, Garcia suggests repeating it to key people over several days or weeks. Just do so appropriately. Start with a casual e-mail before an official memo, and don't jump the office chain of command.

RECRUIT A FRIEND TO YOUR CAUSE

Make it personal. People are more receptive to an idea when it's illustrated by a good story, says Melanie Green, PhD, a psychology professor at the University of North Carolina at Chapel Hill. For instance, a University of Southern California study found those watching the TV drama *ER* were 65 percent more likely than others to eat healthfully after watching an episode featuring obese patients with hypertension.

Your Strategy

Tell a tale. If you're trying to interest a friend in your favorite charity, skip the facts and figures and focus on people the organization has helped and their stories of triumph or sorrow. "Most people recognize that poverty is a problem, but when they learn about what a real person actually experiences, it runs deeper," says Green. Keep in mind, too, that real-life accounts are usually harder to dispute than a set of data.

WIN THE BEST POSSIBLE PRICE

Use the 15 to 20 percent rule. Buyers and sellers overestimate how good a deal they're making when it comes to a home, car, or similar item, says a study coauthored by Richard Larrick, PhD, a business professor at Duke University. Most of the time, researchers found, each party had more wiggle room than she thought—and could've used it to save or make more money.

Your Strategy

Lowball up front. If you are the buyer, offer the salesperson 15 to 20 percent less than what you can really afford. "That way, you'll be leaving room for concessions," Larrick says. For instance, if you absolutely can't spend more than $6,000 on a used car advertised at $7,000, try offering $5,100 (15 percent less than $6,000). Next: Explain why this price is reasonable (the car has a limited warranty or few of the extras you were hoping for). Reverse logic follows if you're the seller: Make the initial price 15 percent more than what you'd accept. If you must get $6,000 for your car, offer it for around $7,000—and have reasons why. Remember: Set a realistic limit and have a plan B if you don't get a deal.

FIND YOUR ZEN

Fresh twists on tried-and-true destressors can take you to a new level of calm

Want to find the ultimate in peace and happiness? The key is to make sure you haven't fallen into a relaxation rut. If your usual stress buster isn't soothing your anxiety like it used to, you need to try something new to boost peace of mind. We found five cool variations on popular pastimes that can settle your nerves in record time.

IF YOU WIND DOWN WITH A BATH . . .

Try a natural hot spring.

Move over, Mr. Bubble. It's worth going the extra tension-taming mile to plunge into a natural spring. "Soaking in hot springs lowers levels of the stress hormone cortisol, which reduces inflammation and built-up strain in your ligaments and joints," says Pamela Peeke, MD, MPH, an assistant professor of medicine at the University of Maryland School of Medicine.

Some top spots include Dunton Hot Springs in Colorado, the Hot Springs Resort & Spa in North Carolina, and Ojo Caliente Mineral Springs in New Mexico. For more ideas, visit Trails.com, which has a substantial database of hot springs, including secluded ones that require a hike through the woods.

IF YOU EMPTY YOUR MIND WITH MEDITATION . . .

Try qigong.

Shake up your seated practice with qigong (pronounced chee-gong, which means "energy work"). This active Chinese meditation routine mixes and matches hundreds of fluid, graceful dancelike exercises. By focusing on these repetitive movements and your breathing, your mind pushes aside intrusive thoughts and elicits the body's relaxation response: Your heart rate slows down and blood pressure, adrenaline, and cortisol levels drop.

Classes are often held at YMCAs, gyms, and community or wellness centers. To find a local instructor, go to the National Qigong Association's Web site, nqa.org.

IF YOU WALK OFF A BAD DAY . . .

Try a labyrinth stroll.

These mazelike paths, which date back thousands of years, have grown in popularity, thanks in part to promising research documenting meditation's effects on blood pressure, cortisol levels, and other markers of stress reduction, according to M. Kay Sandor, PhD, an associate professor of nursing at the University of Texas Medical Branch at Galveston.

Labyrinths can be inlaid on church floors, marked by stones in a garden, mowed into grassy fields, or painted on the ground in public parks. Walkers follow a single circuitous route free of wrong turns or dead ends toward the center.

Most courses take about 20 minutes to complete, but Sandor suggests that you go at your own pace. When you reach the center, take as much time as you'd like for reflection, then retrace your steps back out.

Finding a labyrinth is relatively easy: More than 1,000 hospitals, spas, schools, churches, and wellness centers in the United States have installed labyrinths on-site. (You can also search veriditas.org to find one.)

IF YOU REFRESH YOUR SPIRITS BY HIKING . . .

Try geocaching.

A high-tech version of an old-fashioned scavenger hunt, geocaching has become an increasingly popular weekend activity since global positioning system (GPS) signals were made accessible to the public in 2000. Participants log on to a free geocaching Web site to get the coordinates of "caches"—secret stashes of everyday objects hidden across the world.

Any person, team, or organization can set up and monitor a cache according to safe geocaching rules—in fact, there are already more than 650,000 caches scattered around the globe. Each cache is ranked according to the difficulty of the hunt and terrain, so you can choose a trek that matches your fitness level.

Players plug the specific coordinates into a handheld GPS device that guides them as they walk through woods, snowshoe along trails, or hike through mountain meadows. When you find a cache, you can take the trinket out of it and leave a new treasure behind for the next person to discover. Most caches also include a logbook for you to sign and date with a brief description of your journey. Check out geocaching.com to find cache coordinates in your area.

IF YOU DECOMPRESS WITH MASSAGE . . .

Try Reiki.

Japanese for "universal life energy," this bodywork method involves gentle or no touch. Reiki therapists believe that they can channel energy through their hands and transmit it to the patient, promoting balance and healing.

During a Reiki session, which typically lasts between 60 and 90 minutes, you'll lie on a massage table, fully dressed, while the therapist places her hands in various positions around your head, torso, legs, and feet. Studies have shown that Reiki reduces anxiety and blood pressure. To find a local Reiki therapist, contact the International Association of Reiki Professionals (iarp.org) or the International Center for Reiki Training (reiki.org).

fast fact --
200,000: The number of patients and hospital staffers who benefit each year from RxArt

HEALTH HEROES

She helps people heal through art

Before his cancer treatment, a boy sat mesmerized by videos of flamingos projected on a hospital wall. After radiation, he ran back to see the next animal and was delighted to spot a tiger. Contemporary artwork inspires patients and staff in 13 East Coast medical facilities, thanks to New York–based RxArt. Founder Diane Brown, 60, plans to deliver works to other regions in the next 2 years. "The boy watching the animals forgot he was in the hospital," she says. "That's the whole point."

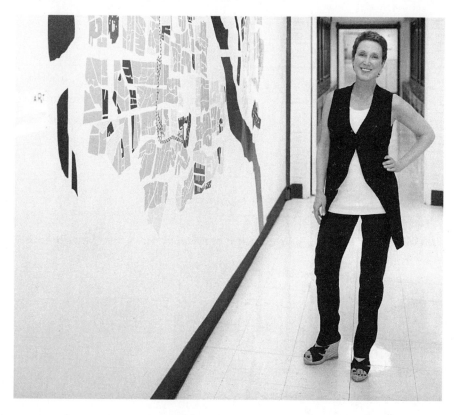

PART

VI

BEAUTY
BASICS

TURN BACK THE HANDS OF TIME

Feel smoother, softer, and younger from the neck down with breakthrough treatments and insider secrets

Father Time is a sneaky little guy. While we're busy working, raising families, and trying to fit in some Must See TV, he's leaving his nasty little calling cards: turkey wattles, spider veins, cherry marks, and more. It's enough to make you want to cover up in your turtlenecks and knit pants all year round. To the rescue: our guide to the latest skin care treatments for every woe from the neck down. Start off with our in-home treatments, and then, if needed, call in the reinforcements found at the doctor's office. In no time, you'll be set to strip off the layers with confidence!

THE PROBLEM: NECK WRINKLES

Years of sunlight can break down the collagen fibers responsible for keeping the skin on your neck looking youthful and firm.

At home: Many skin care creams and lotions smooth the skin, but choose one that includes retinol and peptides. They can build collagen and soften the skin on your neck—even reducing the so-called tree-ring lines. To prevent further wrinkling of the neck, use products with a SPF of at least 15.

In office: In-office options are considered the gold standard, says Ronald Moy, MD, a professor at the David Geffen School of Medicine at UCLA. One to consider: fractionated resurfacing, with lasers such as Fraxel and Affirm. They stimulate cell turnover and the production of fresh collagen by making thousands of microscopic wounds over 20 percent of your skin. Because the surrounding skin is left untouched, the healing time is minimal, and the slight redness it does cause subsides within a few days.

You'll see significant improvement: Fine lines are often reduced by up to 50 percent after five or six monthly treatments at $500 a pop. (Turn to page 287 to read more about Fraxel as a treatment for stretch marks.)

THE PROBLEM: TURKEY WATTLE

As people age, that sharp right angle between the neck and the chin begins to go south. The loss of definition in the neck is due to excess fat, loose skin, and weak muscles.

At home: To reduce sagging, try neck creams that boost collagen production. One of our favorite products is Shiseido Benefiance Concentrated Neck Contour Treatment ($48; Macy's), which contains chlorella extract and hydroxyproline to tighten the skin.

In office: Liposuction performed under local anesthesia is a quick fix, says Yael Halaas, MD, a facial plastic surgeon in New York City. During the half-hour procedure, which costs around $2,500, small incisions are made behind the ears or below the chin; excess fat is vacuumed out via tiny suction tubes. To reduce bruising and swelling, which can last up to 2 weeks, another option is ultrasound-assisted lipo, which employs sound waves that liquefy fat before it's suctioned out. (With either treatment, you'll need to wear a neck sling for 2 weeks to help skin re-drape properly.) If you have excess skin, you may need to pair lipo with a neck lift to completely regain firmness. During the 1- to 2-hour procedure, which costs about $1,000 more, small incisions are made behind your ears or under your chin and then excess skin is trimmed, lifted, and sutured into place.

THE PROBLEM: SUNSPOTS

Those brown spots on your hands and arms can scream 60, even when you're only 40! UV exposure damages pigment-producing cells (melanocytes), causing brown spots to form. "Among drivers, the left hand—the one the sun hits—often looks older," says Kimberly Butterwick, MD, a La Jolla, California, dermatologist.

At home: Use a lotion that contains 2 percent hydroquinone (HQ), the most effective bleaching agent. "HQ works inside the melanocytes to suppress production of melanin, the pigment that makes up this discoloration," says Mary Lupo, MD, a clinical professor of dermatology at Tulane University School of Medicine. Start now. It could take months to notice a difference. For speedier results, choose one that also contains retinol or alpha-hydroxy acid, which helps drive HQ into the skin.

To prevent new spots, sunscreen is key. Use a product that contains a broad-spectrum sunscreen of at least SPF 15. For the best protection, check the label for avobenzone (aka Parsol 1789), Mexoryl, or Helioplex.

In office: Intense pulsed light therapy, or IPL, uses high-intensity pulses of light to target brown spots without harming the skin's surface. You'll need three to five sessions to erase brown spots, with each treatment costing from $500 to $1,000 a pop.

THE PROBLEM: BULGING VEINS

What makes veins on the hands look so inflated? As we age, sunlight breaks down collagen in our hands. As that slight cushion of fat begins to thin, hands start to look skeletal and the veins become more prominent. "Veins that normally wouldn't be visible under plump skin become prominent with collagen and fat loss," says Lee Schulman, MD, an NYC-based phlebologist.

At home: Moisturizers with ingredients that build collagen, such as retinoids, alpha-hydroxy acids, and peptides, can help plump skin so veins stand out less. You don't need a special hand cream, though. "If you're using a product that contains these ingredients on your face, apply it to your hands," suggests Dr. Butterwick. For best results, use an Rx retinoid such as Renova or Avage. To minimize the color contrast between your skin and the purple vessels, apply an opaque concealer or use self-tanner. Other fixes: jewelry and manicures. In one study, people thought women were younger when their hands were adorned with polish and rings. Also, keep your nails short. The white tips should be about 1/8 inch long. "Shorter nail shapes soften the appearance of pronounced knuckle joints and veins," says Jan Arnold, cofounder of Creative Nail Design, a nail care company.

In office: Sclerotherapy is commonly used to treat visible veins on the hands. (For information on sclerotherapy for spider veins, see page 288.) The enlarged veins are injected with a solution that causes them to collapse; blood from those veins is redirected to veins deeper in the hands. Just make sure your budget is prepared: The total treatment, which can involve three to five visits, costs around $3,300.

THE PROBLEM: KERATOSIS PILARIS

Rough, bumpy skin on the backs of your upper arms, butt, and thighs is the hallmark of this very common—and completely harmless—condition. Although keratosis pilaris (KP) looks like tiny pimples, it's actually a buildup of dead cells around individual hair follicles, says Dr. Lupo. A chronic problem that can be treated but not cured, KP frequently—and inexplicably—improves during the summer months and sometimes even gets better as you age.

At home: Regular use of a body scrub, which sloughs dead cells from the skin's surface, can help rub out the problem within a couple of months. To keep follicles from replugging, use a lotion with an exfoliator such as retinol, salicyclic acid, or alpha-hydroxy acid daily, suggests Anne Chapas, MD, an assistant clinical professor of dermatology at New York University School of Medicine. Look for one that's also formulated with urea, a moisturizer that softens the toughest of skin.

In office: Microdermabrasion, a treatment that uses tiny particles to lightly sandblast the top layer of skin, leaves you noticeably softer and smoother. You'll see a significant improvement in KP after two or three weekly treatments, which run about $280 each. If residual redness persists, intense pulsed light therapy may help destroy the redness that creates the polka-dot effect. Each treatment costs $500 to $1,000, and you'll probably need at least three sessions. The pain is bearable, and any subsequent irritation fades within a few days.

THE PROBLEM: CHERRY SPOTS

Good news: These bright red spots (cherry hemangiomas, in medical speak) are harmless. Bad news: They tend to grow in number and size with age—though they rarely become larger than a pencil eraser. Exactly what causes cherry spots, a proliferation of capillaries that commonly appear on the chest, stomach, and back, is a mystery, says David Duffy, MD, a clinical professor of dermatology at the University of Southern California. They are, however, thought to be hereditary.

At home: There's no effective over-the-counter (OTC) treatment for cherry spots, but concealer can help camouflage them. Dr. Duffy recommends using a heavy-duty opaque cover-up, such as Classic CoverMark ($22; covermarkusa.com). If your skin tone is fair to medium, applying self-tanner or dusting on bronzer can also reduce the color contrast between the spots and your skin.

In office: A dermatologist can zap away cherry spots—wherever they are on the body—with the pulsed dye laser (PDL), which zeros in on blood vessels to knock out redness. Although you'll shell out $100 to $300 a PDL session (two or three are recommended), the results are worth it: In one study, cherry spots improved in 97 percent of those treated, and 14 percent saw their spots vanish entirely. Expect some slight stinging and minimal bruising that lasts a few days.

THE PROBLEM: STRETCH MARKS

Like a rubber band that eventually snaps when pulled too far, stretch marks occur when the skin is extended to the breaking point. Usually the

70 to 90: Percentage of women who are plagued by unsightly stretch marks

result of a pregnancy or dramatic increase in weight, the unsightly streaks appear when collagen (which supports the skin) and elastin fibers (which provide elasticity) break apart. Technically considered scars, stretch marks—which most frequently appear on the abdomen, hips, and breasts—initially look pink or purplish and may be slightly raised. With time, they usually assume a thin, sunken appearance and fade to white.

At home: If you're already using a prescription retinoid cream such as Renova to reduce wrinkles, it may help ever so slightly to dab some on your stretch marks as well—especially if they're less than 6 months old. "Retinoids help form new collagen and elastin, which can make stretch marks more similar in appearance to your normal skin," says Dr. Duffy. According to a University of Michigan Medical Center study, 80 percent of patients with fairly new stretch marks treated with a retinoid cream for 6 months saw the length of their marks decrease by an average of 14 percent and the width by 8 percent. You can also try retinol, the less-potent retinoid available in OTC cream. "It's definitely worth a try, but the best results are seen on newer stretch marks," says Dr. Duffy.

In office: Consider a Fraxel laser treatment to stimulate collagen production. In a study of 18 patients conducted by NYU's Dr. Chapas, five Fraxel treatments at 2- to 3-week intervals were found to fade even old stretch marks by about 50 percent. The laser works by emitting a very thin beam of infrared light that makes thousands of microscopic wounds over only 20 percent of your skin—the surrounding tissue is left untouched. This "fractional" approach allows the skin to heal much faster than if the entire area were treated at once, says Roy Geronemu, MD, a clinical professor of dermatology at NYU Medical Center. It also means that side effects—including pain—are minimal. Mild swelling and redness subside in a few days. The drawbacks: Each treatment costs about $500, and up to five sessions are necessary to see optimal results.

THE PROBLEM: SPIDER VEINS

These weblike clusters of red, blue, and purple streaks, each about the width of a hair, affect about 50 percent of women. Spider veins, or telangiectasias, are dilated capillaries that become visible because they're situated so close to the skin's surface. Although the exact cause is unknown, risk factors include hormonal changes from menopause and trauma to the skin, such as bruises. Women who spend a lot of time on their feet are prone to getting them (the pressure on the legs forces the capillaries to fill with blood), as are those who habitually cross their legs or are even a few pounds over their ideal body weight.

At home: DIY solutions include covering spiders with heavy-duty concealer (a quick fix if you only have a few to hide) or applying self-tanner to minimize the contrast between your skin and the colorful vessels. To prevent them, avoid prolonged periods of standing or sitting. Another smart move: wearing tight-fitting support stockings, which decrease pressure that accumulates throughout the day.

In office: A dermatologist can exterminate spider veins with a simple "lunchtime" procedure called sclerotherapy, during which a solution is injected into the vein via a very fine needle. The solution irritates the lining of the vessel, causing it to swell and stick together and eventually collapse in this closed position. Over a period of weeks, the vessel turns into scar tissue that's absorbed by the body, becoming barely noticeable or invisible. Although not an instant fix, sclerotherapy—which doesn't require anesthesia—usually clears 80 percent of spider veins in three or four monthly treatments, says Dr. Duffy. Discomfort is minimal and includes some stinging at the site of injection and possible muscle cramping that subsides after about 15 minutes. Cost: $350 to $750 per session, depending on how many squiggles you have.

THE PROBLEM: INGROWN HAIRS

After shaving or waxing, the curly hairs in your bikini area sometimes get trapped inside the follicle or grow back into the surrounding skin, causing painful, red, pimplelike "bikini bumps."

SIX THINGS TO KNOW ABOUT LASER HAIR REMOVAL

Looking to banish hair for good? Keep these things in mind.

LASERS WORK BEST ON DARK HAIR AND LIGHT SKIN. The light is attracted to color, so it won't be as effective on white, gray, blonde, or red hair. The treatment is most effective on the bikini line and underarms.

"The average woman has coarser, thicker, darker hair in those areas, and that's what is needed to be highly successful," says Deborah S. Sarnoff, MD, a clinical associate professor of dermatology at NYU Medical Center.

YOU NEED MULTIPLE TREATMENTS. Hair cycles between two dormant phases and a single growing phase, and only hairs in the growing phase will be receptive to the laser's zap. As more hair grows in, you'll need additional treatment—usually at least one a month for 5 months. Studies show that a series can reduce hair counts by up to 75 percent, with results lasting as long as a year or more before a touch-up is necessary.

YOU DON'T GET INSTANT RESULTS. "It can take a week to 10 days for treated hair to fall out," says Dr. Sarnoff. Unlike waxing, you don't have to grow out hair for several weeks prior to lasering. A little stubble is all that's needed to attract the light.

IT CAN HURT. The treatment's gotten less painful thanks to cooling tips on the laser and the use of topical anesthetics, but it can still feel like rubber bands snapping your skin.

THERE CAN BE SIDE EFFECTS. The most common are changes in pigmentation, either a lightening or a darkening of the skin. To minimize risk, have the treatment done by a physician or physician-supervised technician, advises Dr. Sarnoff.

IT'S STILL NOT CHEAP. Prices have dropped considerably over the years, but you can expect to pay an average of $500 for the upper lip or chin to $1,500 for the bikini line.

At home: Gentle use of a body scrub or washcloth every other day will help dislodge trapped hairs and prevent their return. For a chronic case, try a product such as Tend Skin, which contains an exfoliant that keeps bumps at bay by eliminating the dead cells that hinder hair from growing out of the skin. Then dab on a pimple medication containing benzoyl peroxide or salicyclic acid to reduce inflammation and stave off bacteria that cause infection, says Cindy Barshop, owner of Completely Bare, a New York City–based spa that specializes in hair removal.

In office: If ingrown hairs become infected, ask your doctor for a prescription-strength antibiotic lotion to kill bacteria and a steroid cream to quell swelling and redness. If you're especially prone to bikini bumps, consider laser hair removal, which makes them a thing of the past.

CHAPTER 34

SUPPLEMENT YOUR SKIN CARE

Pills to smooth skin and strengthen
nails are popping up everywhere.
Here are four that have science
on their side

Are you taking an inside-out approach to beauty? You know that nourishing your mind, body, and spirit enhances your natural glow; what's surprising is that scientists now say it's worth adding supplements to your diet, exercise, and skin routine. "It's important to also feed the skin internally," says Leslie Baumann, MD, director of cosmetic dermatology at the Miller School of Medicine at the University of Miami. "In addition to eating a healthy diet, certain supplements can provide a constant supply of essential nutrients."

Here's the latest on which pills have been scientifically proven to help deliver firmer, more radiant skin and healthier nails.

TO HELP PREVENT AGING

Heliocare: Nothing wears out skin like UV exposure, which is why applying sunscreen is the most important thing you can do to safeguard it. But bolstering skin's UV defenses with Heliocare—a potent antioxidant that mops up free radicals produced by the sun—is a good second step. Derived from a South American fern, the supplement has a huge dermatologist fan base: One loyal user, New Orleans dermatologist Mary Lupo, MD, a *Prevention* advisor, calls it "a slam dunk." "I'm positive it helps," she says. "On a recent trip to Cancún, my husband and I both used sunscreen and took Heliocare one day, and neither of us burned. The following day, we both used sunscreen, but only I took Heliocare—and he burned."

There's strong scientific support for the supplement's skin-protecting ability: It dramatically reduced the incidence of sunburn as well as damage to collagen and elastin, the fibers that keep skin smooth and firm, in two published Harvard Medical School studies. That's because Heliocare is particularly effective against the "aging" UVA rays that most sunscreens don't protect against completely.

Your Rx: Dr. Lupo recommends taking one capsule 30 minutes prior to sun exposure if you're prone to sunburn. If you plan to spend an extended period of time in the sun, take another capsule 3 hours from the first ($60 for 60 capsules; heliocare.com).

FOR SOFT, SMOOTH SKIN

Omega-3 fatty acids: These supplements aren't just making headlines for preventing heart disease. Dermatologists are recommending them to help heal dry skin and the rough, red, scaly patches of psoriasis and eczema. "Countless studies show that increasing the consumption of omega-3 oils improves these conditions," says Dr. Baumann. In one study published in the *British Journal of Dermatology*, volunteers with severe dermatitis taking high levels of omega-3s (6 grams) saw a 30 percent decrease in symptoms. Psoriasis sufferers experienced similar results in other research.

It's easy to see why omega-3s are crucial to skin health: Besides being an integral part of the membranes that surround our skin cells, these essential fats—which must be obtained from diet or supplements because our bodies cannot make them—are a key component of the lubricating layer that keeps skin supple. They also aid in the production of hormones that improve skin texture and help combat the inflammatory damage wrought by free radicals—one of the causes of wrinkles and blotchiness. This is likely why sun-sensitive people may be significantly less prone to burning after omega-3 supplementation, according to one study.

Your Rx: Eating fish such as salmon, mackerel, and albacore tuna—good sources of omega-3s—twice a week and taking supplements are easy ways to increase your intake. For better skin, Dr. Baumann recommends taking 1,000 milligrams of omega-3 oils a day—about the same dosage recommended to keep your ticker in good shape. Try Nordic Naturals Omega-3 Purified Fish Oil ($27 for 120 soft gels; nordicnaturals.com) or Kirkland Signature Fish Oil ($9 for 400 soft gels; costco.com).

TO BOOST FIRMNESS AND HYDRATION

Imedeen Prime Renewal: The idea that a biomarine-based complex can shore up aging skin may sound a little fishy, but the evidence is impressive, says Dr. Baumann. Postmenopausal women taking the supplement (which is recommended for those age 50 and up) saw significant improvement in skin firmness and smoothness in a 6-month study in the *European Journal of Clinical Nutrition*. The results were seen on the face, décolletage, and hands.

Likewise, in a similar 12-week study on women taking a sister supplement (Imedeen Time Perfection, suggested for women 35 to 50), skin's moisture content increased by 30 percent. Other changes include a visible reduction in fine lines, a fading of sunspots, and an overall brighter complexion.

The contents of the capsules—which contain a proprietary protein derived from a deep-sea fish and high concentrations of antioxidants such as vitamin C and lycopene—work in part by increasing production of collagen and elastin, as well as hyaluronic acid, the body's natural moisturizer, says Imedeen's Lars Lindmark, PhD.

Your Rx: Take the Imedeen supplement suggested for your age, advises Dr. Baumann, who uses Time Perfection herself and recommends it to patients. Although a 90-day supply of Prime Renewal ($245) is significantly more expensive than Time Perfection ($180; both at imedeen. us), it supplies twice the amount of the biomarine complex.

FOR STRONG, PRETTY NAILS

Try biotin. Age-weakened nails may have met their match in this B vitamin. Several studies, including one published by dermatologist Richard K. Scher, MD, a professor of clinical dermatology at Columbia University, show that daily supplementation with 2.5 milligrams of biotin significantly improves nail strength—translating into firmer, harder nails that are less likely to crack or chip. (Another possible benefit that

BANISH BRITTLE NAILS

Brittle nails don't mean neglected nails. In fact, sometimes it means quite the opposite. An overzealous manicure can weaken nails and invite infections. Here are some tips to strengthen your nails.

Be sure to always file your nails in one direction with a soft emery board to avoid breakage.

- Never cut the cuticles. They act as a barrier against infection-causing bacteria.
- Soak your nails in warm water to soften the cuticles, and then gently push them back with an orange stick. Use a cuticle nipper to snip away hangnails.
- Don't use old nail polish. Most lacquers made prior to 2007 contain dibutyl phthalate, which is a chemical shown to cause birth defects in rodents.

fast fact --
**25: Percentage taking the B vitamin biotin whose nails grew stronger
in one study**
----

hasn't been studied is thicker hair, which a number of people have reported.) Experts don't know why megadoses of biotin help fortify fragile nails. The idea originated with veterinarians, who give it to horses to harden their hooves.

Although getting nutrients from your diet is most desirable, you'll probably need a supplement to notice a difference in your nails: Eggs and liver, two rich dietary sources, deliver a scant 25 and 27 micrograms (or 100 times less than the studied amount), and many multis provide just 30 micrograms.

Your Rx: Look for a supplement such as Appearex ($25 for a 12-week supply; appearex.com) that contains 2.5 milligrams of biotin. Because the vitamin is water-soluble, it won't build up in the body and cause side effects. To be safe, Dr. Scher recommends checking with your physician before taking biotin and discontinuing use if you haven't seen any improvement at all after 3 months.

long way toward softening fine lines within a few months. But alas, a do-it-yourself routine is nowhere near as fast—or as effective—as what doctors can do.

In this detailed report, you'll get the real scoop on the wrinkle fixers you've always wondered about (Botox), their newfangled cousins (fillers, lasers, and some innovations that are just hitting the market), and why some old standbys (chemical peels) are still worth your while. Prepared with the help of top dermatologists and plastic surgeons, this chapter is loaded with insider tips and expert advice to help you determine the right way to reclaim your skin.

BOTOX

Fixes crow's-feet, forehead furrows, and lip lines

Results: Lasts up to 4 months with little to no downtime

Cost: $380 per treated area

Overview: Botox injections interrupt nerve impulses to the muscles used to squint, frown, and purse the lips. When these muscles relax, fine lines and wrinkles smooth out. According to a review of studies, patients who received Botox felt they looked about 5 years younger. It may take 2 weeks for Botox to kick in the first time. The smoothing effect persists for up to 4 months. Repeat shots tend to take effect sooner (in as little as 2 days) and last longer.

"After being in a relaxed state for so long, your muscles retrain themselves to stay that way," says David Bank, MD, a dermatologist in Mount Kisco, New York. If used early enough (ideally, in the late thirties and early forties), Botox prevents deep wrinkles from setting in.

Ouch factor: Mild stinging. "The needle is only slightly thicker than a hair, and it takes less than 10 minutes to completely treat any of these areas," says Dr. Bank. There's no downtime; you can get 'toxed during lunch, and no one will be the wiser.

Risks: The low dosage levels used in a standard cosmetic injection—25 to 75 units—aren't toxic. (A lethal dose for humans is approximately

IRON OUT YOUR WRINKLES

Lines? What lines? From Botox
and fillers to lasers and peels,
here's how to erase every line—
and love your age

Many things improve with age, but sadly, your skin isn't one of the
Over the years (and after a lifetime of sun exposure), skin often loses
elasticity and resiliency, giving way to wrinkles. Some of you don't m
these lines: In a Prevention.com poll, about 4 percent of responde
declared their wrinkles to be a badge of honor. At the other end of
spectrum, though, is the clear majority—the 57 percent who panic at
sight of their wrinkles in bad lighting.

Like lots of you, we suspect, many of them are getting ready to emp
the big guns to erase the remnants of an unhealthy past. Luckily,
never been easier to eradicate the lines and wrinkles that make you
(and feel) older than you actually are. The right at-home regimen—inc
ing retinoids, peptides, alpha-hydroxy acids, and sunscreen—can

3,000 units.) Reports that link Botox to serious adverse reactions, including 16 deaths, stem from high dosages to treat serious medical conditions. The most common—but still rare—side effects of Botox when used cosmetically are slight bruising that lasts for a few days, a headache, or a strange feeling of heaviness. You may temporarily end up with an uneven brow or a droopy lid if the wrong muscle is targeted or equal amounts aren't used on each side of the face.

Maximize results: Activate the injected muscles for 30 to 60 minutes after treatment—so, for example, squint your eyes as much as you can after having your crow's-feet treated. "That way, more of the toxin will be taken up into the nerve that supplies the muscles," says Jean Carruthers, MD, a clinical professor of ophthalmology at the University of British Columbia. But don't massage the area for 24 hours or the Botox may migrate into unintended neighboring muscles.

FILLERS

Treats "smile" lines, marionette lines, lip lines, and deep lines that Botox doesn't uncrinkle

Results: Lasts up to 6 months; causes bruising for up to 10 days

Cost: $580 per treatment area

Overview: Hyaluronic acid fillers such as Restylane, Juvéderm, and Elevess are smooth gels that instantly fill up wrinkles; HA's ability to attract up to 1,000 times its weight in water helps keep skin plumped. Repeated treatment means longer-lasting effects because injections stimulate new collagen that "lifts" skin.

"After a couple of years, patients often don't need further injections or need less filler to achieve the desired effect," says Dr. Bank. Juvéderm isn't proven to have the same collagen-boosting effect, but experts believe it does. Elevess, the most recently approved hyaluronic acid, lasts as long, or even longer, than other HA fillers.

Ouch factor: Mild to moderate. Despite the use of ultrafine needles, "some patients find it uncomfortable, especially around the mouth," says Kenneth Beer, MD, an assistant professor of dermatology at the University of Miami. Ice, topical anesthesia, and nerve blocks significantly reduce the pain. Elevess is laced with the anesthetic lidocaine, so it causes less pain at the injection site than other HA fillers.

The treatment takes less than 30 minutes but often causes bruising and swelling—so schedule treatments well ahead of important events. Avoid vitamin E, St. John's wort, ibuprofen, aspirin, and other anti-inflammatories for 7 to 10 days prior to treatment to reduce side effects. Sleeping with an extra pillow or two the night you've been injected minimizes swelling, says Dr. Beer.

Risks: A lumpy feel or asymmetry occasionally occurs if the material clumps in one place instead of diffusing evenly. Massage or injection of an enzyme that dissolves HA usually corrects the problem.

Maximize results: HA fillers are malleable, so avoid rubbing the treated areas for 24 hours. Minimizing facial movements in injected areas for several hours also keeps the material in place.

LASER RESURFACING

Significantly improves fine lines and blotchiness

Results: Skin looks badly sunburned for 2 days

Cost: About $1,130 per treatment with fractionated lasers

About $400 per treatment with intense pulsed light (IPL)

About $100 per treatment with light-emitting diode (LED)

Overview: There are many different types of lasers used to rejuvenate the skin. Fractionated lasers, the latest laser technology, emit very thin beams of infrared light that make microscopic wounds over only 20 percent of your skin, triggering the body's natural healing process and accelerating the production of collagen and new, healthy skin cells. One study reported a 25 to 50 percent improvement in lines around the eyes and mouth following 3 monthly treatments with Fraxel, one type of fractionated laser. Where these lasers really excel, though, say some experts, is at wiping out brown spots and blotchiness. Pigment-producing cells are injured during treatment, so they pump out less melanin. It takes 3 to 6 months from your last treatment to see the final results, which last at least 2 years. But noticeable wrinkle smoothing and improvement in discoloration is possible after several sessions.

"That doesn't mean every line will be erased," says Elizabeth Tanzi, MD, a dermatologist in Washington, DC, and a clinical instructor at the Johns Hopkins School of Medicine. "Sometimes you have to use the laser in combination with other treatments like Botox and fillers." Best candidates have mild to moderate sun damage.

Another type of laser resurfacing called intense pulsed light (IPL)

INSTANT FACE LIFT

Bump back time by sporting a ponytail! "It instantly gives your face a lift—softening fine lines and accentuating your features," says Sean James Decuers, a stylist at the Rita Hazan Salon in New York City. To keep your hair healthy, wear yours higher, lower, looser, or tighter from one day to the next. This will prevent breakage and thinning that ponytails can cause.

employs a broad wavelength of light to target brown spots and red areas, destroying them without damaging the upper layers of the skin. Four to six monthly sessions should be enough to even out your complexion; a maintenance session every 6 to 12 months keeps up the results.

Light-emitting diode, or LED, treatments uses light energy to minimize fine lines, reduce pore size, diminish dark spots, and give skin a smoother texture. There's no downtime: You sit in front of a panel of 2,000 tiny pulsing lights for up to 40 minutes; results become more noticeable after 3 weeks.

"LED thickens the skin, so it looks more luminous when light bounces off it," says David Goldberg, MD, a clinical professor of dermatology and director of laser research at Mount Sinai School of Medicine. A study published in the *Journal of Drugs in Dermatology* also showed that the device promotes new collagen formation and decreases inflammation that causes collagen to break down. Six monthly treatments and twice-yearly touch-ups are recommended.

Ouch factor: The newer Affirm and Active FX fractionated lasers are mildly painful, if at all, so an anesthetic is optional; a fan also cools skin to minimize discomfort. Fraxel penetrates the deepest and can be more painful, so docs apply a numbing agent. Downtime is minimal: "You can usually be treated on Friday and be back in commission, with makeup, on Monday," says Dr. Tanzi. LED treatments are painless.

Many doctors are using a topical anesthetic called Pliaglis Cream to reduce the discomfort of laser resurfacing and other cosmetic treatments. A combo of two painkillers, Pliaglis goes on like a cream and dries to an easily removed peel—eliminating the mess of most preparations. In one study, more than 90 percent of laser resurfacing patients had no pain or slight pain when skin was prepped with Pliaglis.

Risks: Complications such as scarring and loss of pigmentation are extremely rare when the procedure is done by an experienced physician.

Maximize results: Use a retinoid and antioxidant for 2 weeks before treatment to speed healing, says Robert Weiss, MD, president-elect of the American Society for Dermatologic Surgery and associate professor of dermatology at the Johns Hopkins School of Medicine. "When skin is softer, you can go deeper with the same amount of energy to deliver a better outcome."

PEELS

Dramatically improves most signs of facial aging (fine lines, deeper wrinkles, and brown splotches)

Results: Requires about a week of recovery time

Cost: Average cost is a budget-friendly $720, or up to $500 per session for lower-strength peels

Overview: During a chemical peel, doctors paint a 25 to 35 percent trichloroacetic acid on the face like a mask to create a controlled exfoliation. Because TCA delves fairly deeply into the skin to remove layers of damaged tissue and stimulate collagen production, you'll need to hide out for a week while you heal. But it's worth it: "Within 7 to 10 days, you'll have a youthful, glowing complexion with noticeably reduced signs of sun damage," says Yael Halaas, MD, a facial plastic surgeon in New York City.

"Decades of studies have shown that you'll see a 50 percent improvement in all but the deepest lines around the mouth," says Dr. Bank. The rejuvenating effect lasts several years.

Ouch factor: Fairly high—at least briefly. For the 2 minutes it takes the acid to neutralize, you'll experience a terrible burning pain, says Mary Lupo, MD, a clinical professor of dermatology at Tulane University School of Medicine. To minimize discomfort during the 45-minute procedure, docs peel the face in sections and cool it with a fan. They may also prescribe oral pain meds.

There's no pain post-peel, but skin feels like it's been badly sunburned. It takes a solid week to recover, and you'll be self-conscious in public. By day 7, at least 90 percent of skin has peeled off, and you can cover the residual pinkness with makeup. If a "vacation" is impossible (or you're squeamish about the recovery), consider having a series of lower-strength

(15 to 20 percent) TCA peels, which produce 3 days of fine, dandrufflike flaking. Three 15 percent peels over several months deliver close to the same results as one higher-strength peel, says Dr. Bank.

Risks: The darker your skin, the higher your risk of complications such as skin discoloration and scarring. Proper aftercare, including keeping skin cleansed and moist, helps prevent the scabbing and infections that can lead to complications.

Maximizing results: Continue to use a home-care regimen—ideally, a retinoid at night and a broad-spectrum sunscreen with SPF 15 or higher daily—to see sustained improvement.

CHAPTER 36

DEFY YOUR AGE

Which skin care products really help
turn back time? We asked a team of
top derms to test the promising new
antiagers. Here are the nine that
deliver results you can see

A staggering number of products are launched every year, each claiming amazing skin-saving benefits. To find out which really work, we did something no other magazine has ever dared to do: enlist leading dermatologists to scientifically test the 45 most promising eye creams, night creams, skin peels, sunscreens, and more. Each product was tested by a group of five women over age 40 for up to 6 weeks—long enough to deliver on its claims. Experts employed state-of-the-art equipment such as the Visia Complexion Analysis machine to accurately determine the winner in each category. This high-tech device compares testers' skin before and after to show improvement in everything from spots and pores to wrinkles and redness. We're pleased to say that judges and testers saw real age-defying results with these nine winners.

BEST EYE CREAM

Priori Smoothing Eye Serum ($60; prioriskincare.com)

Testers gave this serum a chorus of "ayes." "It's wonderful. I've actually gotten compliments on how much younger I look," says one, who reports fewer fine lines and less puffiness and darkness. This doesn't surprise us: Compared with creams, which usually contain less than 10 percent of active ingredients, serums have up to 70 percent, and this one packs no less than a dozen de-agers, including lactic acid (an alpha-hydroxy acid that polishes skin by sloughing dead cells), glycerin and sodium hyaluronate (humectants that attract moisture to firm skin), caffeine (to reduce puffiness), and acetyl hexapeptide-8 (a muscle-relaxing peptide that smooths fine lines).

The serum's pleasant smell, velvety texture, and quick absorption also garnered raves. Light-refracting mica and silica particles instantly soften imperfections. Genius.

Use it right: Apply every other night as directed until skin is acclimated, then use nightly. "Eye creams with AHAs can be drying," says judge William Philip Werschler, MD, an assistant clinical professor at UCLA School of Medicine. They can also make skin more sun sensitive, so use a high-SPF (15 or more) broad-spectrum sunscreen in the morning.

BEST NIGHT CREAM

Peter Thomas Roth Un-Wrinkle Night ($110; peterthomasroth.com)

Talk about a dream cream! This powerhouse rejuvenator refines texture, increases hydration, boosts firmness, and enhances radiance. "Everyone noticed improvement in fine lines after just 2 weeks, and the benefits got even better over time," says judge David Bank, MD, a dermatologist in Mount Kisco, New York.

The quick results come courtesy of a plethora of proven antiagers, including exfoliators such as collagen-stimulating peptides, moisture magnets such as shea butter and glycerin, retinol and glycolic acid, and protective antioxidants such as vitamins C and E. Although retinoids and

AHAs can be drying, no tester—including those with sensitive skin—experienced irritation. In fact, one of the most surprising findings was an improvement in redness, which Dr. Bank attributes to anti-inflammatories such as aloe and allantoin.

Use it right: Apply it to your face and neck after cleansing (avoid the more sensitive eye area), and allow 15 minutes for the rich cream to completely absorb before your head hits the pillow. To avoid deactivating the ingredients, don't use any other leave-on product over it. If your skin doesn't become irritated, boost its benefits with a weekly at-home peel or microdermabrasion treatment. Maintain your results by protecting your skin during the day with a high-SPF (15 or more) broad-spectrum sunscreen.

BEST MICRODERMABRASION TREATMENT

Prescriptives Instant Gratification Skin Renewal Peel ($45; prescriptives.com)

A radiance home run! Testers universally give this product glowing marks for speed and effectiveness. "My skin immediately felt and looked softer and smoother," says one. Another reported benefit: tighter pores. A peel and microdermabrasion treatment in one, the product employs salicylic acid, acetyl glucosamine, and a blend of natural exfoliators mixed with spherical beads to loosen and slough away dulling dead cells to boost brightness.

An added bonus: the relaxing warming sensation that softens skin, increases blood flow, and enhances penetration for faster results, says judge Mary Lupo, MD, a clinical professor of dermatology at Tulane University School of Medicine.

Use it right: Apply at night and use sunscreen in the morning. If skin is normal to oily, use weekly, increasing to twice a week as skin becomes acclimated, says Dr. Lupo. Apply weekly or every 2 weeks if skin is especially dry or sensitive. If your regimen includes AHAs, vitamin C, or retinoids, wait until skin adapts to these antiagers before trying this product.

BEST FACIAL SUNSCREEN

Neutrogena Age Shield Face Sunblock SPF 55 ($10; drugstore.com)

With its silky texture, this facial sunscreen seemed more like a high-priced moisturizer to some testers. "It smoothed my skin and absorbed quickly, so makeup didn't slip and slide as I applied it," reports one converted sunscreen-phobe. Oil free and nongreasy, it didn't clog pores or lead to breakouts, which testers also loved. What's more, this potent sunburn blocker contains Helioplex, a complex that provides strong protection against age-accelerating UVA rays, says judge David Goldberg, MD, a clinical professor of dermatology at Mount Sinai School of Medicine. The formula also features antioxidants to boost skin's built-in defenses. "I wore it on vacation and didn't get sunburned, which I usually do!" contributes another tester.

Use it right: "Applying sunscreen is key to keeping skin youthful, so never skip a day," says Dr. Goldberg. Wear this as your everyday moisturizer (tint it by adding a dab of foundation), or save it for high-sun-exposure days. Don't skimp: Allow a quarter-size amount to shield your face, neck, and chest.

KITCHEN CURE

Broccoli could be sprouting up in your antiaging regimen. Applying a smear of an extract found in broccoli sprouts to skin reduced inflammation and redness—key measures of future skin cancer risk—by nearly 40 percent, according to researchers at Johns Hopkins University School of Medicine. The compound, rich in the antioxidant sulforaphane, activates skin's own cancer-fighting ability by boosting production of protective enzymes. Once stimulated, the mechanism works for days, long after the extract is washed away, says lead researcher Paul Talalay, MD, a professor of pharmacology and molecular sciences. Keep an eye out for topical broccoli-based sun-protective products, which are in development.

BEST LIP TREATMENT

Avon Anew Clinical Plump and Smooth Lip System ($25; avon.com)

This innovative two-sided click pen features a lip plumper on one end and a wrinkle smoother on the other. "My lips instantly looked fuller and smoother," says one tester. A host of hydrators attract water to the lips and surrounding area, adding volume and easing vertical lines that lead to lipstick feathering, says Dr. Werschler. Tingly peppermint oil increases blood flow to temporarily make lips appear poutier and restore their natural healthy color, he adds. Meanwhile, retinol slowly reverses tissue loss that causes the lips to start shrinking in your twenties.

Use it right: First, apply the plumping treatment onto lips and allow it to sink in before using a balm or lipstick. Then coat the area around your lips with the smoothing concentrate. Be patient: It takes a few months to see the final result.

BEST BROWN SPOT FADER

DDF Discoloration Reversal-Pod ($70; sephora.com)

Testers raved about how well this targeted treatment evens out skin tone. "After a month, my brown spots became less noticeable, and my skin looked great without makeup," says one. Ingredients such as n-acetyl glucosamine and niacinamide lighten brown spots by blocking the key enzyme involved in the production of melanin, the pigment that colors skin, and by inhibiting its transfer to skin cells. Niacinamide, a B vitamin, also increases luminosity.

"It usually takes months to see improvement with pigmentation, so the fact that this faded discoloration even minimally so quickly is impressive," says judge Helene R. Rosenzweig, MD, an assistant clinical professor at UCLA School of Medicine. The pod's spongelike applicator, which gently exfoliates skin, speeds results by allowing active ingredients to penetrate skin faster.

Use it right: "If you're not going to be diligent about UV protection, don't even bother using this. You'll re-pigment within moments of sun exposure if you don't wear sunscreen," says Dr. Rosenzweig. Testers wore a broad-spectrum SPF 30 sunscreen daily. Use it day or night; let it dry completely before applying moisturizer or sunscreen.

BEST REDNESS REDUCER

Clinique Redness Solutions Daily Relief Cream ($39.50; clinique.com)

This cream was the hands-down favorite among testers with flushed faces because of dryness, sensitivity, or conditions such as rosacea. Besides reducing ruddiness, it delighted testers with how well it softened and smoothed skin minus the irritation that often accompanies antiagers. Thank the time-released salicylic acid, which gently and gradually exfoliates skin, and heavy-duty hydrators such as shea butter, cholesterol, and linoleic acid, says judge Ranella Hirsch, MD, president of the American Society of Cosmetic Dermatology and Aesthetic Surgery. Other star ingredients include anti-inflammatories such as bisabolol; glycine; a complex of white, yellow, and red tea; and antioxidants such as green tea, vitamin E, and resveratrol. What's not in the cream is also important: fragrance and the most common preservatives, which can inflame sensitive skin.

Use it right: The product doesn't contain sunscreen, so some testers preferred to use it at night. "It's a little heavy under sunscreen," notes one. That may be a plus when skin is parched or temps and humidity levels are low. But in an either/or situation, opt for sunscreen. "UV exposure is a common trigger for redness," says Dr. Hirsch.

BEST BODY SUNSCREEN

Aveeno Continuous Protection Sunblock Spray SPF 70 ($9.50; drugstore. com)

This sunscreen scored top marks for its light scent, high SPF (no one from our Southern California panel of testers ever burned!), and ease of application. The bottle sprays upside down, making hard-to-reach spots more accessible, and the clear formula doesn't have to be rubbed in with your hands. (Research shows that sunscreen use increases dramatically with easy-to-use sprays, and testers were uniformly consistent with daily application.) Other key skin-saving benefits: strong, long-lasting protection against aging UVA rays from stabilized avobenzone, and built-in antioxidants such as vitamins A, C, and E that offer extra insurance against UV exposure, according to Dr. Rosenzweig.

Use it right: To protect against day-to-day UV exposure, spray on exposed areas at least 20 minutes before heading outdoors. "Don't wait until you're already outside. By then the damage will have begun," says Dr. Rosenzweig. If you're going out for an extended period of time, liberally cover skin before dressing, and reapply every 2 hours or immediately after swimming or toweling dry.

BEST DAILY MOISTURIZER WITH SPF

Vichy Laboratoires UV-Activ Daily Moisturizer Cream with Sunscreen (SPF 15) ($29; vichyusa.com)

Testers were so enamored with this elegant everyday lotion that one stocked up on two more bottles before running out of the first! "It's no surprise this product scored so high," says judge Arielle Kauvar, MD, a clinical associate professor at New York University School of Medicine.

For starters, it's wonderfully hydrating due to glycerin, a humectant that plumps up fine lines by attracting water to skin. It also contains Mexoryl, the best blocker of "aging" UVA rays. But besides preventing future damage, the antioxidant-rich moisturizer proved it can also reverse signs of aging—Dr. Kauvar detected a decline in testers' sunspots. "Studies show that regular use of sunscreen repairs skin," she says. Bonus: Unlike most day lotions that take time to "set," this lightweight formula absorbs so fast that you can apply your makeup right away. What's not to love?

Use it right: Apply in the morning to your face and the oft-neglected neck and décolletage at least 20 minutes before heading out the door. Keep in mind: "This product isn't sweat or water resistant, so it's not suitable for extended sun exposure," says Dr. Kauvar.

To find a customized routine for your skin type, go to Prevention.com/perfectskin.

BANISH BREAKOUTS FOR GOOD

Derm-tested solutions, breakthrough
treatments, and the latest science
to keep your complexion
blemish free and beautiful

It's a cruel irony that more than half of adult women are battling break-outs at the same time they're coping with crow's-feet. Contrary to popular belief, greasy foods and dirt do not cause acne. The culprit is hormones, which ebb and flow throughout a woman's life rather than stabilize as they do in men.

"As estrogen levels fluctuate—or in the case of menopause, decrease—androgens, the hormones that stimulate oil glands, can lead to break-outs," says Jonette E. Keri, MD, PhD, an assistant professor of dermatology at the University of Miami School of Medicine. The progestin found in many birth control pills can also aggravate acne. Greasy hair, skin products, perspiration, headbands, and other things that can plug up pores tend to make acne worse. Also to blame: stress, which raises hormone levels.

One thing you needn't stress about is controlling the condition. New remedies make it easier to get the clear skin you've always wanted—and erase signs of aging in the bargain.

BEAT BLEMISHES AT HOME

The following skin care routine fights the main cause of acne: pores clogged by oil and cellular debris and inflammation from *P. acnes* bacteria. But unlike topical teenage treatments, which are formulated for oilier complexions, these over-the-counter solutions are less likely to dry mature skin and make wrinkles more pronounced. (Read above to find out which products we like best.) The routine relies on treatments that address the dual concerns of acne and aging by employing the following agents.

Salicyclic acid, which unclogs pores and smooths skin by sloughing off dead cells.

Retinoids such as retinol, a vitamin A derivative that improves acne, fine lines, and sunspots by normalizing cellular turnover.

Humectants that attract moisture and anti-inflammatories, including green tea and allantoin, to quell inflammation.

Follow the following steps to eradicate pimples and prevent new one.

In the Morning . . .

Cleanse gently. Use a facial wash with salicylic acid. "It gets into the pores and dislodges debris," says Diane Berson, MD, an assistant professor of dermatology at the Weill Medical College of Cornell University and board member of the American Acne and Rosacea Society. Avoid gel cleansers, which might contain alcohol, and granulated scrubs, which strip the skin oils, making it overcompensate and produces even more, says Dr. Keri.

Treat affected areas. If you have a blemish, dab on a spot corrector with salicylic acid or benzoyl peroxide, which kills surface bacteria and dries oil. If you're prone to breakouts in a particular area (say, your chin), apply it to the entire zone daily to help prevent them.

If skin is dry, apply a moisturizer with SPF 15 or higher. Choose one that contains an alpha-hydroxy acid such as glycolic acid for an added

---

CLEANSE WITH CARE

When using facial cleansers—especially foaming or gel types—always apply them to damp skin. When cleansers are used on dry skin they are more likely to cause irritation. And to make sure you're giving your cleanser a fair shot at wiping out pollutants, dirt, and bacteria, gently massage the face wash into your skin for about 1 minute before rinsing it off.

double benefit: The AHA exfoliates pores as it sloughs off dead cells and
moisturizes skin.

If your complexion is oily, use an oil-free sunscreen. UV rays
tend to thicken the outer layer of the skin, which can, in turn, block pores
and lead to breakouts.

At Night . . .

Remove makeup with a gentle, nonmedicated cleanser. The skin
can't exfoliate properly if it's not clean.

Apply a retinol cream. The prescription retinoid Retin-A was
approved for treating acne long before it became the gold standard for
fighting wrinkles. "Retinoids help clear up and prevent all kinds of acne,
from tiny bumps and blackheads to inflammatory acne and red nodules
around the jawline," says Dr. Keri. Over-the-counter retinoids like retinol
don't pack the same punch as Rx versions, but they can be less irritating
and a good way to acclimate skin.

Moisturize when needed. Apply moisturizing lotion to your face frequently to prevent dryness.

WHAT YOUR DOC CAN DO

If your skin doesn't respond to at-home treatments within a few weeks or
if you have you have many pimples (especially cystlike nodules, which are
large, painful, and can cause scarring), see a dermatologist. She'll prescribe a more potent retinoid and topical antimicrobial such as benzoyl
peroxide to kill bacteria and quell inflammation.

Bonus: New Rx meds are more appropriate for aging and dry skin. "If
there's not enough improvement after a few months, other drugs can be

added," says Dr. Berson. The following are also available in a dermatologist's antiacne arsenal.

Oral antibiotics: A 2- to 6-month course speeds healing by targeting deeper blemishes. These drugs travel through the bloodstream, so they also fight hard-to-reach back and chest acne.

Hormone therapy: To steady hormones and quiet premenstrual flares, patients are often put on a low-dose birth control pill. One caveat: Women who are over 40 can be at increased risk of developing the same side effects associated with hormone therapy to reduce menopausal symptoms, including blood clots. Also prescribed in conjunction with oral contraceptives or by itself is spironolactone, which is an antiandrogen that decreases oil production.

Light therapy: These treatments are used in conjunction with other Rx remedies to boost their benefits. Blue light therapy temporarily kills *P. acnes* in a painless 15-minute procedure. The bacteria can return, however, so ongoing therapy—at up to $500 a pop—is necessary.

The new Isolaz Pore-Cleansing Acne Treatment suctions your pores to eliminate excess sebum, while a laser targets the bacteria. Four to six sessions (costing $300 to $500 each) are needed, followed by monthly maintenance sessions.

For additional smooth skin solutions, you can check out Prevention. com/clearskin.

KITCHEN CURE

One possible way to stay pimple free is to avoid eating refined foods such as white bread and pasta. Recent Australian research finds that this fare pumps up production of the hormone androgen, increasing oil production. "Bacteria on the skin break down the excess oils, irritating hair follicles, which triggers breakouts," says Jennifer Linder, MD, a clinical instructor of dermatology at the University of California, San Francisco.

GET A LOCK ON HAIR COLOR

Get head-turning hair color at home with these foolproof formulas and easy pro tips

There's nothing like a great dye job to look younger, fast. On the other hand, going gray can be profoundly liberating! No matter what your tress preference is, you can put your hair in the trusty hands of these experts who explain the new do-it-yourself rules for beautiful color tones.

DYE IT YOUR WAY

Hair color not only covers the gray, but it also boosts volume and shine, makes fine lines less noticeable, and brightens a dull complexion. That is, unless you're still coloring the same way you did in your thirties. "What worked then might be aging you now," says Kim Vo of the Mirage Las Vegas. Here are the rules you should follow to make you look and feel a decade younger (no salon required!).

Choose an Age-Defying Shade

Extremely light or dark hair looks harsh against mature skin. For the most youthful effect, lighten hair about two shades from your current natural color (for instance, from medium brown to light brown or dark blonde; dark blonde to medium or light blonde), while selecting a cool or warm undertone that complements your skin.

"Going lighter softens your face, so fine lines and age spots look less noticeable," says Gary Howse, creative director of Seattle's Gary Manuel Salon. Besides being more flattering, it also minimizes the possibility of mistakes and avoids noticeable roots.

Go Multi-Tonal

The vibrancy of youthful hair comes from the subtle contrast of color—a mix of highlights and lowlights against your base color. "Nothing is more aging and looks more unnatural than hair that's flat and all one color," says Brad Johns, Clairol's global color director. Here are two easy ways to recreate this radiant effect

Use a multi-tonal dye. Both demi and permanent formulas of this type feature a combination of dye molecules that mimics the nuances of younger hair—dark strands will be deepened and grays washed into lighter glints. A tip-off that a dye delivers multidimensional color: The product name contains words such as shimmering, blended, or tone-on-tone. To hide a smattering of silver, choose a demi-permanent dye; if you're more than 40 percent gray, opt for a permanent color.

Add highlights. If you want more visible contrast than a multi-tonal dye delivers, frame your face with a few strategically placed highlights. Bonus: These winning streaks make eyes look brighter and give skin a healthy glow.

"Go two to three shades lighter than the rest of your hair," says Mary Button, a colorist at Philadelphia's Adolf Biecker Salon. Opt for a warm shade to compensate for skin sallowness; look for words such as golden, honey, or amber in the product's name. Stick with hues that are closer to your hair color; for example, brunettes use light brown, not blonde, and redheads use copper.

SALON-WORTHY COLOR AT HOME

Try the quality tools for a professional-looking hair color.

FOR SHINE: The silicone in Fekkai Salon Glaze ($28; Sephora) allows you to make your hair gleam.

FOR HIGHLIGHTS: Ammonia-free Revlon Frost & Glow Highlighting Kit ($9; drugstores) creates subtle or dramatic streaks with less damage.

FOR BLONDES: With specially formulated dyes, UV filters, and conditioners, L'Oréal Paris Superior Preference Dream Blonde Complete Color & Care System ($15; drugstores) neutralizes harsh hues to keep blondes bright.

FOR EXTRA DIMENSION: Available in six permanent shades, Garnier Color Breaks ($7.30; drugstores) can be used immediately postcoloring to add lighter or darker tones.

FOR QUICK RESULTS: A fast-acting lightener in Clairol Perfect 10 by Nice 'n Easy ($14; drugstores) delivers permanent color in 10 minutes—reducing hair's exposure time to harsh chemicals by 50 percent.

Remember, less is more: Aim for about 10 quarter-inch streaks on each side, beginning about ⅛ inch back from your face and spaced ½ inch apart until just past your ears. Perfect your technique by "sketching" your pattern beforehand with conditioner, which has a similar consistency to hair color.

Apply Like a Pro

For foolproof home coloring that delivers salon-worthy results, try the following tips.

Concentrate on your roots. When we're younger, our hair is naturally lightest at the ends. To recreate this effect, apply dye to your roots, but not your ends (as some kits instruct). They soak up color the fastest because they're so porous. During the last 3 minutes of processing, splash water onto the crown of your head and then comb color through from top to bottom.

"That shot of water dilutes the dye, creating a more natural-looking hue," says James Corbett, owner of James Corbett Studio in New York City. Rinse hair until water runs clear. Then apply the kit's conditioning treatment, and rinse well. Wait at least 24 hours before shampooing.

Employ heat. Because heat opens the hair's cuticle, warming an old towel in the dryer and wrapping it around your head after applying the dye allows the formula to soak into gray's more stubborn hair shaft.

Try a gloss. There's now a host of at-home glosses (once only available at salons), including tinted formulas that help intensify a fading shade. "They contain silicones that coat and smooth the cuticle, allowing light to reflect evenly," says Vo. Use monthly to maintain shine and vibrancy.

Go Out with a Bang

Bangs are the age-defying 'do. "They cover crinkly foreheads and reduce the appearance of crow's-feet by focusing attention on the eyes," says Travis Speck, a stylist at Bumble and Bumble in New York City. When cut correctly, they also frame your face, restoring definition to your cheeks, brows, and eyes. If your face is round, consider a cut with layered wispy pieces that graze the tops of your brows. If you have a square face, wear bangs long and side-swept to soften angles. And if your face is long and thin, add blunt bangs that fall just above the brows to give the illusion of fullness.

THE WAY TO GRAY

Wash that gray right out of your hair? More of you are saying "No way!" According to L'Oréal, nearly half of women over age 40 are no longer hitting the bottle. Besides being practical (no more pesky roots!), going gray makes a statement of supreme confidence: This is who I am, and I'm proud of my natural beauty.

It can also look pretty darn fabulous: Think Meryl Streep's chic silver cut in *The Devil Wears Prada*, Jamie Lee Curtis's stylish silver pixie, or

FIVE TIPS FOR STERLING SILVER

The following top-notch products will keep your silver gleaming.

FOR MANAGEABILITY: Used weekly, Clairol Nice 'n Easy ColorSeal Conditioning Gloss ($4; drugstores) has safflower oil to control coarse strands.

FOR SOFTNESS: Non-color-depositing Pantene Pro-V Silver Expressions Conditioner in Sterling to Snow ($6; drugstores) smooths hair without tinting it blue.

FOR BEATING BRASSINESS: The chamomile-derived azulene in Phyto Phytargent Whitening Shampoo (24$; beauty.com) helps remove yellowing residue.

FOR SHINE: The luminosity-enhancing silica and rice bran oil in Aveda Brilliant Emollient Finishing Gloss ($23; aveda.com) takes tresses from dull to dazzling.

FOR MAINTAINING MOISTURE: Daily washing and styling can dry out hair; by absorbing excess oils, Bumble & Bumble Hair Powder in White ($19; for salon locator, see bumbleandbumble.com) lets you skip a day or two. (Spray powder directly onto scalp and brush out excess.)

Emmylou Harris's stunning salt-and-pepper mane. Still, if you want to give gray a try, you'll need to know how to avoid the awkward growing-in stage that occurs when you stop dyeing your hair; the mere thought of clashing incoming and outgoing tones keeps many women from returning to their roots. But fear not; these step-by-step rules will help you look terrific every minute of the way to gray.

Go Gradually

Wait until your roots are at least 60 percent silver before giving up your dye job, so your new hue will look symmetrical and natural as it grows in, suggests colorist Jennifer J., owner of Juan Juan Salons in Beverly Hills, California. But don't give up color altogether just yet. "The contrast in texture and tone as your hair grows can look unkempt," she notes. During this phase, which can last up to a year, get a do-it-yourself highlighting kit or ask your colorist to weave in a few fine highlights or lowlights (darker streaks) to add dimension and blend in the roots.

Consider a New Cut

Cropping your hair above your collarbone during the in-between period will lessen the contrast between silver and pigmented strands. Layers can also help camouflage multiple hues.

GET TO THE ROOT OF THE PROBLEM

If regular touch-ups fail to keep your tresses looking youthful, then perhaps you need to look a little deeper. When hair looks dull and frizzy, it could be that your scalp needs some TLC. Keep your hair healthy with a weekly 5-minute scalp massage. This will boost blood flow and feed nutrients to follicles for optimal growth. Also, protect your scalp and hair by wearing a tightly woven hat when going outside for extended periods of time.

"A choppy cut looks youthful and helps hide your roots," says Jonathan Gale, a colorist at the John Frieda Salon in Los Angeles. When your gray has grown out, don't regress to a matronly 'do. "For gray to look glamorous and chic, your cut should be contemporary," says Mark DeVincenzo, creative director at the Frédéric Fekkai Salon in New York City. To enhance silver strands, which absorb light, making your mane look dull, style hair straight (use a flatiron or a dryer and a round brush) to promote shine. Once your hair is completely white, talk to your stylist about adopting an above-the-shoulder, layered style that provides movement and softly frames your face.

Pick Silver-Specific Products

When hair turns gray, the protective cuticle thins out, which can make strands coarse and prone to breakage. Keep tresses soft and healthy by doing the following.

Moisturize. Choose a moisturizing shampoo to soften and smooth hair and make it appear more lustrous.

Prevent yellow. Wash hair with a formula geared for gray once a week to counteract yellowing caused by sun, pollutants, hard water, and smoke. But don't overdo it: Many of these products contain a blue tint that can cause a purplish cast.

Gloss over. Apply a clear gloss or glaze monthly to coat the cuticle and boost shine.

Choose clear. Opt for gels and mousses that are clear: The dyes in colored stylers can tarnish gray hair.

PEER INTO A BEAUTIFUL FUTURE

Innovations to make you look as young as you feel

You may feel like you're at war with your wrinkles each and every morning when you look into the mirror, but actually the battle against those age-old problems like sagging skin and skimpy lashes is being waged—and won—in the scientific laboratories of cosmetics manufacturers. From a high-tech DIY device that reprograms aging skin to an ingenious treatment to help you get a younger-looking wink, here on the following pages are the latest giant leaps for womankind—and exciting new promises for tomorrow.

AN ADDITIVE THAT PROTECTS SKIN

Chelators are topical chemicals being infused into skin care formulas in an effort to remove iron, which is an essential nutrient that gives us energy but is a menace to our skin health.

How is it that iron—which is found naturally in skin in what's known as a safe "bound" form—takes such a big toll on skin? Blame the sun. When iron is exposed to UV light, it becomes unbound. This in turn causes the release of massive amounts of free iron in cells.

"This free iron triggers the production of harmful free radicals that can damage collagen and cause DNA mutations—ultimately leading to skin aging and even cancer," explains Charareh Pourzand, PhD, a lec-

ON THE CUTTING EDGE

Get younger-looking skin with these five innovative remedies created by top derms.

SLOW SKIN AGING. Use Dr. Brandt Lineless Tone ($40; Sephora) after cleansing; chamomile soothes skin while green tea protects against damaging free radicals.

LOOK WELL RESTED. Besides moisturizing delicate tissue, Skin Effects by Dr. Jeffrey Dover Dual Action Under Eye Therapy ($20; CVS) also contains Eyeliss, an ingredient that reduces puffiness.

ERASE BROWN SPOTS. The vitamin C in Murad Essential-C Daily Renewal Complex ($90; Sephora) suppresses the dark pigment melanin to help fade splotches.

SMOOTH WRINKLES. With the muscle relaxer GABA, Patricia Wexler M.D. Advanced No-Injection Wrinkle Smoother ($29.50; Bath & Body Works) eases expression lines.

MINIMIZE SAGGING. When applied topically, peptide- and retinol-packed Rodan + Fields Anti-Age PM Serum Night Treatment Capsules ($75; rodanandfields.com) boost collagen to help fight gravity.

For more derm-developed picks, go to Prevention.com/dermskincare.

turer in pharmaceutics at the University of Bath in Great Britain.

Chelators bind to and isolate the iron so it can't wreak havoc on the skin. Pourzand, who recently published a study on the subject in the *Journal of Investigative Dermatology*, is testing a new product that employs these ingredients. Meanwhile, Dennis Gross, MD, an associate clinical professor of dermatology at New York University Medical Center, has already added a chelating complex to several of his MD Skincare product line.

"While this chelator sequesters the free iron, it still allows the absorption of bound iron, which is beneficial to the healthy functioning of skin," he explains. Though his offerings contain the first topical chelators, expect to see more products formulated with them.

"Adding chelators to skin care products means better skin protection," says Janet Blaschke, a cosmetic chemist in Manhattan Beach, California.

Where to get it: mdskincare.com, including Hydra-Pure Oil-Free Moisture ($75) and Powerful Sun Protection SPF 30 Sunscreen Packettes ($42)

A SERUM THAT SPEEDS SKIN REPAIR

Remergent's DNA Repair Formula is the first skin care product to tackle past DNA damage from UV exposure, which is a major cause of aging. The serum, which is applied to the face twice daily, uses marine and botanically derived enzymes to enhance skin's natural DNA-repair mechanism.

Minimizing DNA damage is key to keeping skin smooth and firm. That's because DNA, the master control for all cellular functions, directs skin cell regeneration. Left untreated, damaged DNA alters the genetic code of cells, causing them to lose their ability to function—and paving the way for fine lines, brown spots, and possibly skin cancer. Although our skin contains enzymes that rebuild DNA, they work slowly, taking a full 24 hours to mend only a fraction of the UV damage.

"The body's natural ability to repair itself may not be enough," explains Daniel Yarosh, PhD, the founder of AGI Dermatics, the company that makes Remergent. (A molecular biologist, Yarosh had previously worked at the National Cancer Institute, where he specialized in gene repair.)

The three encapsulated enzymes in the serum seem to boost your natural repair system, pinpointing and patching up damaged DNA. One study showed that it decreases wrinkling and sunspots after a month of twice-daily applications.

"The evidence suggests that this form of DNA repair may be the key to promoting overall skin health," says Ronald Moy, MD, director of dermatology at California Health and Longevity Institute in Westlake Village. Dr. Moy uses the serum himself and recommends it to every mature patient with sun damage. All have seen the effect of overall younger-looking skin. His assessment: "It's one of the most promising skin care products on the market."

Where to get it: remergentskin.com ($125 for a 2-month supply)

A CUTTING-EDGE EYELASH ENHANCER

Eyelash transplant surgery offers hope to people born with skimpy eyelashes—or those who have lost some or all of their lashes as a result of aging, illness, or injury. Now these women, who until recently had only cosmetic solutions, can permanently improve their "batting average."

Surgeons are restoring the look of lush, natural lashes through a process similar to surgery for treating hair loss. They harvest hair from a postage-stamp-size spot on the back of the scalp, isolate individual hair follicles, and implant them into tiny puncture points on the top eyelid. During the 2 to 3-hour procedure, for which patients are awake but sedated, anywhere from 10 to 80 lashes can be transplanted per lid, explains Jeffrey Epstein, MD, a New York City and Miami-based plastic surgeon who specializes in hair-replacement surgery.

"Normal upper lids contain about 100 lashes, but as few as 20 can create an appearance of normality," he says. Because hair on the head is genetically programmed to grow longer than eyelashes, the newly grafted hair needs to be trimmed every few months. Another grooming must: crimping daily with an eyelash curler, so the transplanted hair behaves as eyelashes would. Side effects of the surgery, which runs about $3,000 a lid and isn't covered by insurance, include short-term soreness, swelling, and itching.

Where to get it: To find a doctor in your area, check out the International Society of Hair Restoration Surgery at ishrs.org.

A TOOL THAT REPAIRS SKIN DAMAGE AT HOME

GentleWaves, a light-based therapy that employs 2,000 tiny blinking lights (imagine sitting in front of a Lite Brite-like screen), has long been

POWERFUL NEW WAYS TO TREAT WRINKLES

It may be hard to pronounce, but idebenone (eh-DE-be-known) spells younger-looking skin. The antioxidant is small enough to penetrate deep into skin to repair damaged cells, says David McDaniel, MD, an assistant professor of clinical dermatology at Eastern Virginia Medical School. Here's how to reap the benefits.

IN A MOISTURIZER: A time-release formula, Prevage Anti-Aging Night Cream ($125; elizabetharden.com) delivers a steady stream of idebenone to repair skin while you sleep.

IN A PILL: Taken daily, Priori Idebenone Supplements ($60; prioriskincare.com for locations) shield skin from the inside out.

IN MAKEUP: Infused with light-reflecting pigments and idebenone, True Protective Illuminating Concealer ($30; truecosmetics.com for locations) brightens dullness and helps keep skin smooth.

available in doctors' offices for several years. Coming soon: antiaging nirvana—smoother skin, smaller pores, and less noticeable brown spots, in the convenience of your own home.

Unlike lasers and other heat-based therapies that stimulate the skin's repair mechanism by injuring it, GentleWaves and GentleWaves at Home are akin to "loading new 'software' into cells to reprogram them," says David McDaniel, MD, an assistant professor of clinical dermatology and plastic surgery at Eastern Virginia Medical School and a consultant to Light BioScience, which makes the devices. Both work by delivering a patented wavelength, frequency, and dose combination of light. "If aging cells are producing less collagen, we use light energy to fuel them to make more," says Dr. McDaniel.

A multicenter trial of 90 patients using GentleWaves published in the journal *Lasers in Surgery and Medicine* yielded some impressive findings: After eight twice-weekly 60-second treatments, all subjects saw an average increase of nearly 30 percent in collagen production, and 90 percent of them had smoother texture and a reduction of redness, discoloration, and lines around the eyes. More frequent use is said to offer even better results.

The downside: Scheduling regular doctor appointments is time-

KITCHEN CURE

A grapefruit a day may keep fine lines and flaky skin at bay, found a recent study in the *American Journal of Clinical Nutrition*. Researchers discovered that women 40 and older who had greater amounts of C were 11 percent less likely to develop wrinkles.

"Vitamin C boosts collagen production, which keeps skin firm," says lead researcher Maeve Cosgrove, PhD, a nutritional epidemiologist. To ward off wrinkles, consume the RDA of 75 milligrams—the amount found in a grapefruit.

consuming and—at $100 to $150 a pop—expensive. That's why the at-home version of GentleWaves is considered to be a major advancement. "Now women will be able to use light to reenergize their skin on a daily basis," says Roy G. Geronemus, MD, a clinical professor of dermatology at New York University Medical Center. As of now, no one is willing to divulge too many details about the DIY tool. Dr. McDaniel says it might be as small as a lipstick or as large as a bathroom mirror.

Where to get it: Stay tuned to lightbioscience.com to find out when the new GentleWaves gets the go-ahead from the FDA.

CREDITS

PHOTOGRAPHS

Page v and pages 200–202:
©Jonathan Pozniak

Page 11: ©Russell Kaye

Page 39: ©Reena Bammi

Page 73: ©Dave Lauridsen

Page 83: ©Ken Schles

Page 123: ©Greg Miller

Page 133: ©Kevin Miyazaki

Page 173: ©Robert Gallagher

Page 179–181: ©John Kernick

Page 183: Courtesy of
James Burling Chase

Page 188–193: ©Peter Lamastro

Page 231: ©Amanda Friedman

Page 251: ©Joe Toreno

Page 277: ©Grant Delin

ILLUSTRATIONS

Page 203–210: ©Ulla Puggaard

INDEX

Underscored page references indicate sidebars and tables. **Boldface** references indicate photographs and illustrations.

V

Vaccines
  for autoimmune diseases, 6
  cervical cancer, 11
Vaginal infections, 4, 119, 121
Vegetables. *See also specific vegetables*
  for belly fat reduction, 130
  health benefits of, 50
  for hunger control, 146, 147
  keeping peels on, 88
  organic, 113
  slicing, for retaining vitamin C, 88
  for weight control, 139
Vegetarianism, for losing last 10 pounds,
    158–59
Veins, bulging hand, 284
Vichy Laboratoires UV-Activ Daily
    Moisturizer Cream with Sunscreen,
    311–12
Visualization
  during exercise, 221
  for morning energy, 235
Vitamin absorption, healthy fats
    increasing, 86–87
Vitamin B$_{12}$, for improving sleep, 108
Vitamin C, for skin health, 81, 332
Vitamin D
  health benefits of, 22–23, 70–72
  in High-Metabolism Diet, 209
  in pain relief combinations, 47

W

Wagging downward dog, 203, **203**
Waist size, cardiovascular risks from, 15
Wakeup strategies, 233–36
Walk-a-marathon (or half) program, 175,
    181–82, 184, 184
Walking. *See also* Walking workouts
  for calorie burning, 213
  for losing last 10 pounds, 156–57
Walking paths campaign, 183
Walking workouts
  for all-day energy, 236, 237
  motivation for, 177
  6-week fat-blasting plan, 175, 176–81,
    179–81
  walk-a-marathon (or half) program, 175,
    181–82, 184, 184
Water
  for energy during dieting, 106–7
  for hydration, 51–52, 221
  as metabolism booster, 160, 208
  for morning energy, 235
  for skin health, 25
  unclean, campaign against, 123
Water bottles, plastic, health risks from,
    62–63, 62

Watermelon
  for cancer prevention, 80
  storing, 90
Weight, effect of organic foods on, 112
Weight gain
  fiber preventing, 79
  weekend, 139
Weight loss
  after age 40, 135–39
  for belly fat reduction, 130–31
  benefits of, 54–55
  breakfast for, 134
  for cellulite reduction, 185–86, 194–95
  cravings control for, 149–54
  grapefruit for, 63–64
  hunger control for, 141–47
  interval workouts for, 176
  for last 10 pounds, 155–63
  resistant starch aiding, 128, 129
  surgery for, 34
Western United States, health care in, 28,
    30–31
Whole grains, for hunger control, 147
Wine
  for belly fat reduction, 131
  red, preventing Alzheimer's disease, 264
Women's preventive health care, regional
    differences in, 28, 35
Work
  improving concentration at, 244–45
  persuading coworkers at, 270–71
Workouts. *See also* Cardio workouts;
    Exercise; High-Metabolism
    Workout; Interval workouts;
    Walking workouts
Worrying
  about forgetfulness, 266–67
  mind wandering from, 249–50
Wrinkles
  treatments for, 81, 282, 297–304, 328,
    331
  vitamin C preventing, 332

Y

Yoga
  for the forties, 203–4, **203–4**
  for skin health, 26
Yogurt
  for digestion, 80
  good bacteria in, 122
  "Live & Active Culture" seal on, 121
  organic, 114
  as preworkout snack, 99

Z

Zinc, for postworkout energy, 220–21
Zyflamend, for pain relief, 42–43, 47